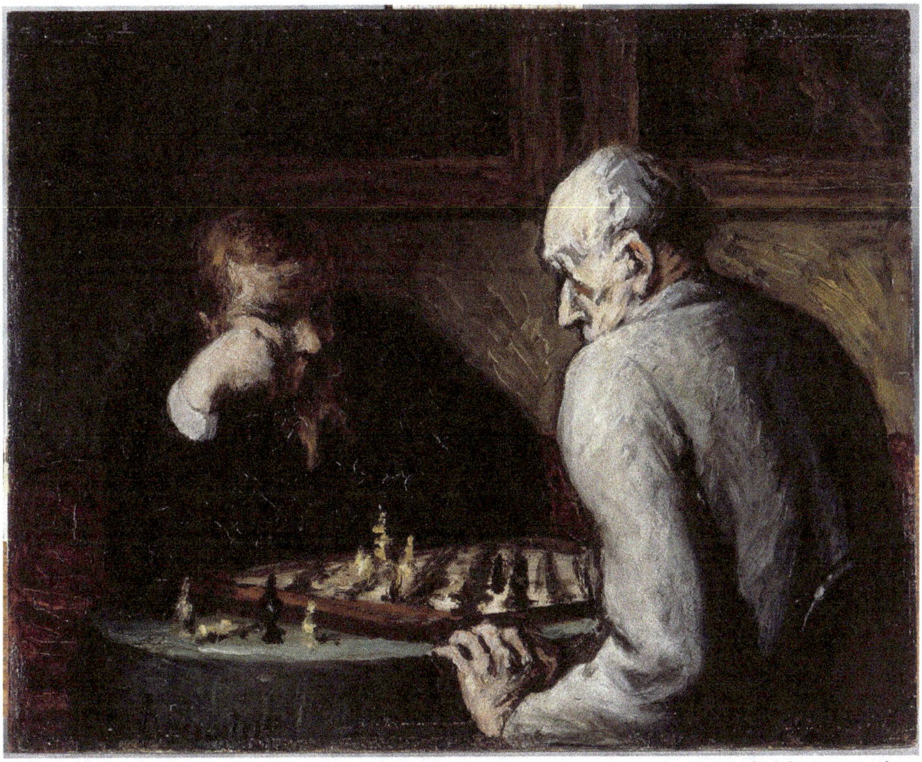

Intellectual activities such as playing chess or regular social interaction have been linked to a reduced risk of Alzheimer's disease in epidemiological studies, although no causal relationship has been found.

FAMILY *and* AIZHEIMER's

Dementia and Alzheimers Disease Treatment

&

How to Prevent Alzheimer's

by

Giulia Rossi

"Caregiving often calls us to lean into love we didn't know possible."
— **Tia Walker**

"Alzheimer's is the cleverest thief, because she not only steals from you, but she steals the very thing you need to remember what's been stolen." — **Jarod Kintz**

PART 1

Introduction

Family and Alzheimer's – The Unspoken Earthquake

When Alzheimer's disease enters a family, it does not arrive as a single patient's diagnosis. It arrives as an unspoken earthquake, its tremors shifting the foundations of every relationship, role, and shared memory. The focus naturally falls on the individual at the center of the storm—the one forgetting names, faces, and routines. But in the shadows, a parallel story unfolds: the story of the family, transformed overnight into a caregiving team, grappling with a profound and disorienting "role reversal."

This is not a journey of a single person fighting a disease. It is the story of a daughter who must now bathe the father who once taught her to ride a bike. It is the story of a husband who must find a way to communicate with the wife who no longer recognizes his face. It is the story of siblings navigating complex medical decisions, financial strain, and the emotional whiplash of grief, guilt, and exhaustion. The most important truth that is often unspoken is this: **Alzheimer's is a family disease.** Its impact radiates outward, touching everyone in its wake, forcing a reconstruction of identity, responsibility, and love itself.

In this guide, we will not shy away from the heartbreak. We will acknowledge the frustration, the loneliness, and the sheer weight of the responsibility. But we will also illuminate the path forward. We will explore how to find moments of profound connection beyond memory, how to build a sustainable caregiving plan that protects your own well-being, and how to navigate the complex emotional landscape as a family unit. This is not about finding a cure for the disease, but about discovering a reservoir of strength, resilience, and compassion you never knew you had. Your family's story is being rewritten, not ended.

How to Prevent Alzheimer's – The Empowered Brain

For decades, the narrative surrounding Alzheimer's disease has been one of fear and fatalism. A diagnosis was often seen as a pre-written fate, a genetic lottery lost. But a quiet revolution is underway in the scientific community, fundamentally changing how we view our cognitive destiny. The most empowering and groundbreaking discovery in modern neurology is this: **Alzheimer's disease is not an inevitable consequence of aging, and our genes are not our destiny.**

While a small percentage of cases are strongly hereditary, the vast majority are influenced by a complex interplay of genetics, lifestyle, and environment. The emerging, powerful consensus is that **what is good for your heart is also good for your brain.** This isn't about a single "magic bullet" pill or superfood. It's about a holistic, proactive approach to building a resilient brain capable of withstanding the challenges of time.

Think of your brain not as a fixed, static organ, but as a dynamic, constantly changing ecosystem. You have the power, through daily choices, to either nourish this ecosystem or poison it. You can plant the seeds of new brain cells, fertilize neural connections, and weed out inflammation. This concept, known as "cognitive reserve," suggests that by building a richer, more connected brain, you create a buffer against the damage caused by diseases like Alzheimer's.

This guide is your blueprint for building that buffer. We will move beyond the headlines and dive into the evidence-based pillars of prevention: the foods that act as medicine, the specific types of exercise that spark brain growth, the sleep that cleanses toxic waste, and the mental habits that forge stronger neural pathways. Prevention is not a destination; it is a lifelong journey of empowered choices. It starts not in a doctor's office, but in your kitchen, on your walking path, and in your daily routines. Your brain's future is, to a remarkable degree, in your hands. Let's begin.

CHAPTER 1 — Understanding Alzheimer's and Its Stages

Why knowledge protects families from fear, confusion, and surprise

Alzheimer's is often described as a disease of memory. But for families, Alzheimer's is really a disease of change. It changes communication, behavior, daily routines, family roles, and long-term plans. When families understand what is happening inside the brain—and what to expect at every stage—they feel less scared and more prepared. Knowledge replaces fear with confidence.

✅What Alzheimer's Actually Is

Alzheimer's is the **most common cause of dementia**, accounting for **60–80% of all dementia cases worldwide**. The number of people affected continues to grow. Today, **more than 55 million people** worldwide live with dementia, and that number is expected to **almost double by 2050**.

Inside the brain, Alzheimer's causes:

- Death of brain cells
- Loss of communication between neurons
- Shrinking of brain tissue, especially memory areas
- Disruption in thinking, judgment, language, and behavior

Most families don't realize Alzheimer's is a **progressive disease** —it keeps changing. That's why early knowledge is a lifesaver.

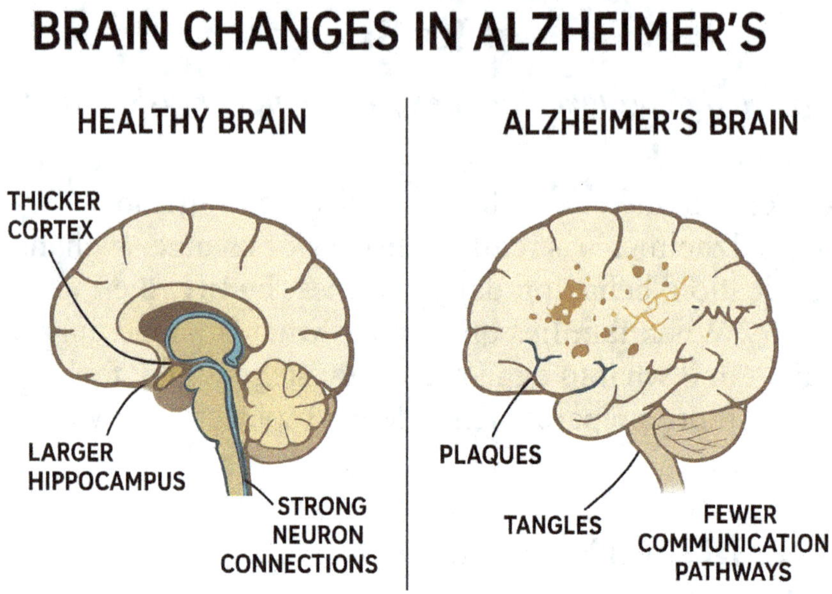

Figure 1: Brain Changes in Alzheimer's

A side-by-side diagram showing:

- Healthy brain: thicker cortex, larger hippocampus, strong neuron connections
- Alzheimer's brain: shrinkage of hippocampus, presence of plaques & tangles, fewer communication pathways

This helps families see the disease is **biological**, not a personality change or stubbornness.

✅The 3 Major Stages of Alzheimer's

There are detailed medical staging systems, but families find these 3 simple stages more useful:

Stage	Cognitive Skills	Daily Life	Common Family Challenges
Early	Forgetful, misplaces	Mostly	Denial,

Stage	Cognitive Skills	Daily Life	Common Family Challenges
	items, repeats questions, trouble finding words	independent	frustration, early conflict
Middle	Confusion, wandering, personality changes, difficulty with routine	Needs help with hygiene, meals, safety	Exhaustion for caregivers
Late	Limited speech, high dependence, bed-bound or chair-bound	Needs full care	Emotional grief, decisions about hospice

✅Story: "We Thought She Was Just Being Difficult"

Maria's mother, age 71, started asking the same question: "What day is your birthday?"
The family laughed at first. "Mom always forgets dates," they said.

Soon, she stopped paying bills on time. She accused neighbors of stealing her purse (it was in the refrigerator), and she started leaving the stove on.

The family argued:

- *"She's getting old—this is normal."*
- *"She's fine, just stressed."*
- *"She's being stubborn."*

One day she wandered outside at night, confused and barefoot. Only then did the family take her to a doctor.

She was diagnosed with early-stage Alzheimer's.

Maria says:

> "If we had understood the warning signs earlier, we

could have protected her sooner. We lost time because we believed myths."

Maria's story is common. Families miss early signs because they expect Alzheimer's to look dramatic from day one. But it doesn't.

✅ MYTHS FAMILIES GET WRONG (And the Truth)

❌ Myth #1: "Memory loss is normal for aging."

✅ **Truth:** Normal aging causes slow recall—Alzheimer's causes losing entire events, names, conversations, and familiar places.
If someone forgets *where they put their keys*, that is normal aging.
If someone forgets *what keys are used for*, that is not normal aging.

❌ Myth #2: "If they can still talk and walk, it's not Alzheimer's."

✅ **Truth:** Alzheimer's begins years before abilities disappear. By the time families see big changes, the disease has already been progressing inside the brain.

❌ Myth #3: "There's nothing we can do."

✅ **Truth:** Families can improve safety, comfort, independence, nutrition, mood, sleep, and communication.
You cannot cure the disease, but you **can change the experience**—and that is powerful.

✅ Chart: Early Warning Signs Families Usually Miss

[Chart: Red Flags Over 12 Months]
A bar chart showing the most commonly reported early symptoms:

- Repeating questions or stories (83%)
- Forgetting appointments (79%)
- Getting lost in familiar places (63%)
- Sudden changes in judgment or spending (58%)
- Personality changes or paranoia (44%)

Most families notice **memory problems**, but don't realize **personality and judgment changes** are also early Alzheimer's signals.

✅The Three Stages Explained for Real Families

Stage 1 — Early Alzheimer's

People hide their symptoms well:

- They joke about forgetting
- They avoid conversations where they might be embarrassed
- They withdraw from hobbies, social events, or driving

Families often think the person is lazy, depressed, or uninterested—not sick.

What families should do:
✔ Get a medical evaluation
✔ Begin organizing legal and medical paperwork
✔ Start routines and visual reminders
✔ Encourage exercise and brain social activity

Pro-Tip #1:
Don't argue or correct every mistake. It creates stress and lowers confidence.
Instead, gently guide without pointing out errors.

Hidden Pitfall:

Families wait too long before involving doctors—losing valuable planning time.

Stage 2 — Middle Alzheimer's

This is the longest and hardest stage for most caregivers.

Common changes:

- Trouble dressing, bathing, cooking
- Mood swings, anxiety, or aggression during confusion
- Repeating questions constantly
- Wandering, especially at night

The biggest danger in this stage is safety—falls, kitchen accidents, wandering, medication mistakes.

Pro-Tip #2:
When a loved one resists bathing or eating, it is not about stubbornness.
Often, they are:

- Scared of water
- Confused by instructions
- Embarrassed about needing help

Changing tone, lighting, or routine can make bathing calm instead of stressful.

Hidden Pitfall:
Families try to handle everything alone.
Burnout becomes dangerous.
This is when respite care, day programs, or helper services are life-saving—not a failure.

Stage 3 — Late Alzheimer's

The brain's communication pathways become deeply damaged.

Signs:

- Limited speech or silence
- Bed-bound or wheelchair-bound
- Difficulty swallowing
- Sleeping much more
- Recognizes faces fewer times, but still feels love and comfort

Families often experience “anticipatory grief”—mourning the loss of connection even before death.

Pro-Tip #3:
Speak gently even if they cannot respond.
Hearing and feeling love remain until the very end.

Hidden Pitfall:
Families assume a loved one is “gone” because they don’t talk. But they often respond emotionally to music, touch, prayer, or familiar voices.

✅What Makes Alzheimer’s Different From Dementia?

Families sometimes confuse the terms:

- **Dementia** is a group of symptoms (memory + thinking + behavior problems).
- **Alzheimer’s** is one **cause** of dementia.

Analogy:
Dementia is like a fever.
Alzheimer’s is one reason someone has a fever.

✅The Hidden Side Families Don’t See: Early Brain Changes

Researchers discovered something surprising:

- By the time the first memory loss appears, the brain has already been damaged for **10–20 years**.

That's why prevention and early evaluation matter.
It's also why families should never feel guilty: the disease began long before signs appeared.

✅ Short, Relatable Story #2 — "The Day We Found the Car"

Jamal's father, age 76, used to drive every morning to the same coffee shop.
One day, he didn't return.
The family panicked. They called neighbors, then police.
His car was found parked miles away, door open, his father confused on a stranger's porch.

Jamal said,

> "We thought we could ignore the memory issues. That day changed everything."

This event didn't mean Jamal's father was "crazy" or "irresponsible."
It meant his **navigation memory**—a part of the brain called the hippocampus—was failing.

✅ Practical Skills Families Can Use Right Now

Problem	What Helps
Repeating questions	Write answers on a whiteboard, keep routines predictable
Forgetting medication	Pill organizers, alarm reminders, caregiver oversight
Wandering	Door alarms, GPS trackers, safe walking spaces
Bathing resistance	Warm towels, calm voice, music, same time each day

Problem	What Helps
Arguments	Redirection, distraction, humor, avoiding correction

Families can transform daily stress by understanding triggers instead of reacting emotionally.

✅"Blame the Disease, Not the Person"

This mindset changes families.

When a loved one:

- Gets angry
- Misplaces items
- Accuses you of stealing
- Says something hurtful

It's easy to take it personally.
But **behavior is a symptom**, not a choice.

Families who learn this early experience less conflict and more compassion.

✅The Most Important Lesson of This Chapter

Alzheimer's is not just a memory disease—it is a communication disease and a planning disease.

Families who learn early:
✔ reduce stress
✔ prevent crises
✔ protect safety
✔ make better decisions
✔ feel more in control

Knowledge is a powerful emotional medicine.

✅ End-of-Chapter Summary

- Alzheimer's affects 60–80% of dementia cases
- It progresses in 3 broad stages: Early, Middle, Late
- Early signs are subtle and easy to ignore
- Behavior changes are biological, not personal
- Families can make life safer, calmer, and happier with preparation
- Knowing what to expect protects everyone

✅ Chapter 1 Reflection Question

What early signs have you seen in your loved one—memory, behavior, or personality—without realizing they may be part of Alzheimer's?

This is a deeply important and personal question. The early signs are often subtle, easily mistaken for normal aging, stress, or just "a phase." Looking back, the puzzle pieces seem obvious, but at the time, they were just confusing, isolated incidents.

Here are some of the common early signs, framed through the lens of what we might have dismissed them as, before we knew.

Memory & Cognition: The "Senior Moments" We Excused
•**Forgetting Recent Conversations:** It wasn't just forgetting a name. It was asking the same question three times in an hour, not remembering a detailed conversation we had the day before. We'd say, "You just told me that," and they'd insist we never spoke about it. We chalked it up to them not listening.
•**Misplacing Items in Illogical Places:** It's one thing to lose your keys. It's another to find the remote control in the freezer, or their wallet in the sugar bowl. We laughed it off as a "funny brain fart."

•**Struggling with Familiar Tasks:** Watching a brilliant cook forget the recipe they'd made for 40 years. Seeing a meticulous person struggle to work the TV remote they'd used for years. We called it "technological confusion" or just being distracted.

•**Losing Track of Dates and Time:** They'd forget what day of the week it was, but so do we all, right? It became a sign when it was constant, when they'd get confused about the season or lose whole chunks of time.

Behavior & Personality: The "They're Just Changing" Shifts

•**Loss of Initiative & Apathy:** They used to love gardening, but now the plants are wilting. They were an avid reader, but the book sits untouched for months. We didn't see it as a symptom; we thought they were just "slowing down" or had lost interest in their hobbies.

•**Increased Anxiety or Agitation in Crowds:** A formerly social person would become visibly uncomfortable and irritable at family gatherings. They'd cling to their spouse. We thought they were just being grumpy or antisocial, not realizing the noise and chaos were now overwhelming and confusing for their brain.

•**Uncharacteristic Mood Swings:** A flash of anger over something trivial. Sudden, unprovoked tears. A generally calm person becoming suspicious or paranoid (e.g., accusing people of hiding things or stealing from them). We took it personally, thinking, "Why are they being so mean?"

•**Withdrawal from Social Life:** They'd make excuses not to meet friends for lunch or skip their weekly card game. It was easier to say "I'm tired" than to admit they were struggling to follow conversations or feeling embarrassed about their memory lapses.

Communication: The "Just a Mental Block" Moments

•**Struggling to Find the Right Word:** This was one of the biggest ones. It went beyond "tip-of-the-tongue." They'd substitute a word with a vague description like "that thing for the thing" or use the wrong word entirely. We'd often jump in to supply the word, thinking we were being helpful.

•**Repeating Stories:** They would tell the same story, word-for-word, in the same afternoon. Unlike the normal repetition of a favorite anecdote, this was new information, repeated as if for the first time.

•**Difficulty Following or Joining a Conversation:** In a group talk, they'd go quiet. They'd lose the thread of a plot in a movie or TV show. We thought they were just bored or not paying attention.

The Heartbreaking Realization:

The moment it clicks is rarely one single thing. It's the pattern. It's when you stop saying, "Oh, that's just Dad being forgetful," and start to feel a deep, unsettling worry that something is fundamentally wrong. The person is still there, but something is subtly shifting behind their eyes.

The key takeaway is this: **If you are noticing a pattern of these changes that is interfering with daily life, it is crucial to talk to a doctor.** Early diagnosis can open doors to management strategies, treatment options, and planning for the future.

CHAPTER 2 — How Alzheimer's Affects the Whole Family

Why emotional, social, and financial preparation is just as important as medical care

When someone is diagnosed with Alzheimer's, the disease does not belong to one person—it belongs to the whole family. Alzheimer's forces spouses to become caregivers, children to become decision-makers, and everyday routines to become unpredictable. Families are loving, but love alone is not enough. Preparation, communication, and shared responsibility are what protect the family's mental health, relationships, and financial stability.

Alzheimer's Is a Family Disease

Studies show:

- **92% of family caregivers** experience high emotional stress
- **1 in 3 caregivers** develop anxiety or depression
- **Nearly 70%** say they feel overwhelmed or alone
- **Over 60%** report conflict with siblings or other family members over care decisions

These numbers show something families rarely admit: **Alzheimer's doesn't break one brain—it breaks family systems** unless people learn how to adapt.

✅ A Relatable Story: "We Thought We Were a Team"

Samira, age 45, lived with her husband and two children. When her father began repeating conversations, losing keys, and forgetting names, the family joked about it. But soon, Samira became responsible for:

- Cooking for both households

- Driving her father to appointments
- Paying his bills
- Checking his medications
- Answering phone calls at work every time he panicked

Her brother lived in another city. He called once a week and said,

> "You're exaggerating. Dad is fine."

Eventually, Samira collapsed from exhaustion. She was admitted to the hospital with severe migraines and high blood pressure.

Her father had Alzheimer's, but **she** was the one ending up in the emergency room.

This story is common. **Caregiver burnout** is one of the most dangerous "hidden injuries" of Alzheimer's.

The 4 Areas of Family Impact

1. Emotional Impact

Families feel a mix of emotions:

- Sadness watching abilities fade
- Stress from constant responsibilities
- Anger toward siblings who don't help
- Guilt for losing patience
- Fear of the future
- Confusion — "Is this normal or part of the disease?"

Even young children feel the changes. Many don't understand why Grandpa forgets them or accuses people of stealing.

Myth #1: "Good families don't struggle."

✅**Truth:** Every loving family struggles. Alzheimer's tests patience, marriage, and mental health. No one is emotionally prepared the first time.

2. Relationship Changes

Alzheimer's changes roles:

- A wife becomes a nurse
- A son becomes a legal decision-maker
- Siblings become business partners managing money, doctors, and care

Most common conflict:
One sibling does all the work, while others stay distant, deny the problem, or only visit on "good days."

Psychologists call this the **"Invisible Caregiver Effect."**

- The person who helps the most is often the most exhausted
- The person who helps the least often believes everything is fine

This imbalance is how families break apart.

Pro-Tip #1:
Create a schedule and shared task list. Even distant relatives can help:

- Pay bills online
- Arrange transportation
- Manage medical appointments
- Check in by phone every evening
- Order groceries or supplies

Not all help requires physical presence.

3. Daily Life Challenges

Families face challenges they never expected:

- Repeating the same answer 25 times
- Middle-of-the-night wandering
- Sudden anger or fear during showers
- Refusing to eat
- Forgetting how to use the toilet
- Asking for deceased relatives

A healthy brain can follow logic and instruction.
An Alzheimer's brain cannot—so arguing never works.

Hidden Pitfall:
Families try to reason with the person:

- "You just ate."
- "We talked about this already."
- "Stop asking me that."

This causes stress.
Instead of arguing, **redirect**:

- "Let's take a walk."
- "Can you help me fold these towels?"
- "Would you like some tea?"

Pro-Tip #2: Distraction is a tool, not disrespect.
It protects dignity.

4. Financial Impact

Alzheimer's care is expensive. Families are often shocked.

Average annual costs:

- **Home care:** $15,000–$40,000 per year

- **Memory care facility:** $45,000–$80,000 per year
- **Nursing home:** $90,000+ per year
- **Adult day programs:** $7,000–$25,000 per year

One family member often:

- Quits a job
- Reduces work hours
- Stops social activities

Caregiving can become a **second full-time job**.

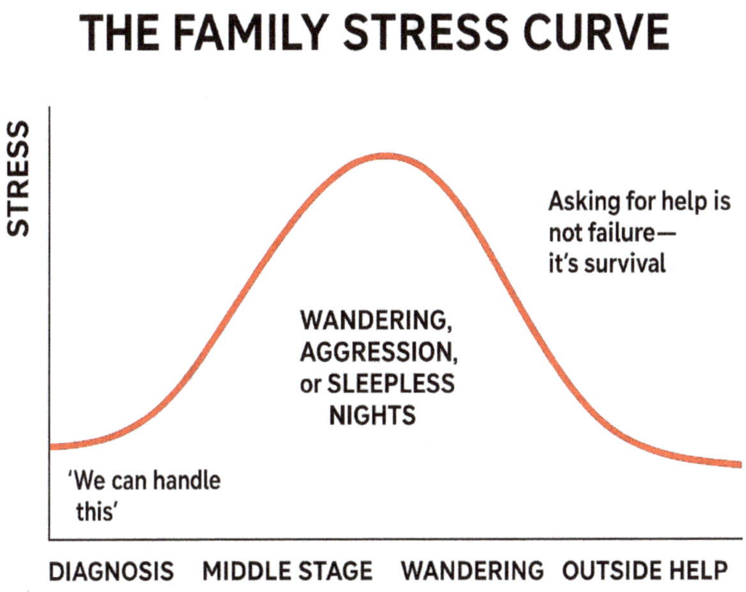

Diagram: "The Family Stress Curve"

A simple line graph showing:

- Stress is low at diagnosis (family thinks "we can handle this")
- Stress rises quickly in middle stage
- Peaks when wandering, aggression, or sleepless nights begin

- Declines only when families get outside help or hospice support

This visual helps families see:
✅ Stress increasing is normal
✅ Asking for help is not failure—it's survival

✅ Another Real Story: "The Day We Locked the Doors"

Hassan, age 76, was calm and gentle. One night, he left the house at 3 AM to "go to work," even though he had retired 10 years ago. His daughter found him walking down the street in slippers.

The next day, the family installed:

- Door alarms
- GPS tracking watch
- Automatic lights in the hallway
- A sign on the front door that read: "STOP. Bathroom is this way."

This was not overreacting—it was **prevention**.

Families fear making their home "feel like a nursing home." But safety is love, not control.

✅ Myths Families Believe (and the Reality)

Myth	Reality
"They are doing this on purpose."	They're scared, confused, or lost. The brain cannot process instructions.
"If we explain it better, they will understand."	Logic doesn't fix a damaged memory pathway. Emotional comfort works better than facts.
"He doesn't recognize me, so he doesn't love me."	Recognition may fade, but emotional memory and safety responses remain. They feel you, even if they cannot name you.

Myth	Reality
"Asking for help means we are weak."	Asking for help means the family survives longer—with fewer injuries and breakdowns.

✅ Pro-Tips for Protecting the Family

✅ Pro-Tip #3: Schedule "Rotation of Responsibility"

Create a weekly or monthly plan:

- One person handles medical appointments
- One manages finances
- One handles meal prep or grocery deliveries
- One stays overnight certain days
- One checks in by phone daily

Caregiving is not fair by itself—**it must be organized**.

✅ Pro-Tip #4: Expect Personality Changes, Don't Fear Them

Alzheimer's can cause:

- Paranoia ("Someone stole my wallet")
- Anger or sudden crying
- Depression or extreme silence

These are symptoms of brain changes, not intentional cruelty.

The family rule:
Blame the disease, not the person.
This protects relationships from emotional wounds.

✅ Pro-Tip #5: Protect Your Marriage and Children Too

Some caregivers focus so hard on their parent that their own household collapses.

- Couples fight
- Children feel invisible
- Financial pressure grows
- Everyone feels resentment

Hidden Pitfall:
The caregiver becomes so busy helping one person that they accidentally ignore the rest of the family.

Take time for:
✔ one movie night a week
✔ a meal together
✔ a walk with your partner
✔ laughter

Rescue the family, not just the patient.

✅The Silent Crisis: Caregiver Burnout

The world talks about Alzheimer's patients.
But very few talk about the caregivers who pay the price.

Signs of burnout:

- Exhaustion
- Crying easily
- Getting angry quickly
- Forgetting your own health
- Losing energy, joy, or patience
- Feeling hopeless
- Feeling alone even in a full house

This is not weakness.
Caregivers suffer because they **care too much and rest too**

little.

Important Statistic:
Caregivers are **63% more likely** to develop serious health problems than non-caregivers.

The Solution: Build a Support Network

Support is not luxury—it's survival.

Sources of help:
✔ relatives
✔ home nurses
✔ adult day programs
✔ neighbors
✔ faith communities
✔ online support groups
✔ respite care
✔ government or nonprofit services

Many families don't know **respite care** even exists:

- Provides short-term care
- Gives the caregiver a break
- Prevents emotional collapse

A tired caregiver is **not helpful**, not safe, and not healthy.
A supported caregiver is a blessing.

The Emotional Journey Families Don't Expect

Families experience:

1. **Shock** — "This can't be happening."
2. **Denial** — "He's just old, it will be fine."
3. **Anger** — at siblings, doctors, themselves
4. **Sadness** — watching the person change

5. **Adaptation** — accepting help and learning skills
6. **Courage** — doing the best they can every day

The most dangerous phase is **denial**.
Denial delays safety, planning, and emotional healing.

End-of-Chapter Summary

- Alzheimer's affects the entire family emotionally, financially, and socially
- Family conflict and caregiver burnout are common, not failures
- Safety planning prevents accidents, wandering, and emergencies
- Asking for help is a sign of intelligence, not weakness
- Protecting the family means protecting everyone, not just the patient

Reflection Exercise

Write down:

- Who is doing most of the caregiving?
- Who can help—even from a distance?
- What task would relieve the most stress if shared?

Who is doing most of the caregiving?
Who can help—even from a distance?
What task would relieve the most stress if shared?

Here are clear, practical answers to those three questions—useful for planning real family support around Alzheimer's care:

1. Who is doing most of the caregiving?

In most Alzheimer's families, **one primary caregiver carries most of the responsibility.**
This is often:

- ✅A spouse (most commonly the wife)
- ✅An adult daughter
- ✅Or in some families, the oldest child or the one who lives closest

Statistics (commonly cited in caregiving research):

- About **60–70% of caregivers are women**
- Roughly **1 in 3 caregivers provide care full-time**
- Over **50%** report high physical or emotional stress because they are doing **too many tasks alone**

Reality check: Even when a family "agrees" to share care, one person typically becomes the default caregiver—often without planning.

Example:
Maya has two siblings. All said they would help with mom's care. Six months later, Maya is doing all doctor visits, medications, bathing, and meals—because she lives closest. She never asked for help directly, and everyone assumed she was "managing fine." But she was burning out silently.

2. Who can help—even from a distance?

Many relatives believe they "can't help" because they don't live nearby—but **distance caregiving is real and very valuable.**

People who can help remotely:

- Adult children who live in another city or country
- Siblings

- Cousins, aunts, uncles
- Grandchildren (teenagers can help with digital tasks!)
- Friends and neighbors
- Church/community groups

Tasks that can be done from anywhere:

Remote helper can…	Why it matters
Order groceries or medications online	Saves hours of errands
Pay bills, manage insurance, paperwork	Removes admin stress
Schedule medical appointments	Gives caregiver mental relief
Call and emotionally support caregiver	Prevents burnout
Arrange housekeeping help	Lifts daily workload
Track medications or reminders by phone	Prevents mistakes
Research resources, therapists, or respite services	Saves time and energy

Important principle:

Even one hour of help per week makes a difference.

People don't help because they don't care—they don't help because they don't know what to do. You must **assign tasks clearly**, not just "please help more."

3. What task would relieve the most stress if shared?

Every family caregiver is overwhelmed by different things, but research shows the tasks that create the **highest burnout** are:

✅**Top stress-relieving tasks if shared:**

Task Shared	Stress Reduced
Bathing, dressing, toileting	High physical & emotional relief
Nighttime care (wandering,	Sleep improves, burnout

Task Shared	Stress Reduced
bathroom trips)	drops
Doctor visits & transportation	Saves time and missed work
House cleaning, laundry, grocery shopping	Daily burden lifted
Managing finances & paperwork	Mental load reduced
Providing weekly respite time	Prevents caregiver depression

If caregivers could choose just ONE shared responsibility, most would choose:

✅ **Respite care—someone takes over a few hours a week**
Even 2–4 hours weekly changes everything.

Simple exercise families can do today:

Ask the primary caregiver these 3 questions:

1. **What is the single hardest task for you right now?**
2. **What would give you back freedom or sleep?**
3. **What task could someone else handle without confusion or training?**

Then assign roles clearly:

✔ "David handles all medications & pharmacy pickups."
✔ "Sarah orders groceries every Monday."
✔ "Uncle Sam calls Mom every night at 7pm to keep her calm."
✔ "Grandkids do laundry and dishes on weekends."
✔ "Sibling in another city manages bills and insurance."

A short story showing how this works

Carla cared for her father alone. She handled bathing, meals, cleaning, bills, doctor visits, and nighttime wandering. She felt guilty asking for help.

One day she made a list of **what stressed her most**:

- Bathing
- Cleaning
- No sleep when her father paced at night

Her sister lived far away, but together they made a plan:

- Sister pays for a part-time aide to help with bathing
- Neighbor's teenager mows the lawn weekly
- Sister calls every evening to keep Dad calm before bed
- Carla gets one full afternoon off every Sunday

✅After 3 weeks, Carla was sleeping again
✅Her father was calmer
✅And the siblings were working as a team

Moral:
You don't need many helpers—you need **specific** helpers.

Quick Pro Tips

✅Don't ask: *"Can anyone help?"*
Instead say: **"Can you handle groceries every Friday?"**

✅Don't wait until burnout.
Ask for help early—**asking for help is not weakness, it's protection.**

✅Even children/teens can help: reading, music, companionship, technology, reminders.

✅If family refuses or disappears, use **community help**: volunteers, senior centers, respite programs, dementia organizations.

CHAPTER 3: Communication and Behavior Challenges

Understanding and Managing Confusion, Anger, Repetition, and Wandering with Calm, Connection, and Safety

When Alzheimer's enters a home, it changes the way people speak, listen, and behave. A person who once handled conversation effortlessly may suddenly struggle to find words, forget recent events, or misinterpret intentions. Family members often describe feeling like they are "talking to a different version" of the person they love.

This chapter breaks down **why behavior changes happen**, what families often get **wrong**, and—most importantly—**how to respond in a way that calms rather than escalates**.

Why Alzheimer's Causes Confusion, Anger, or Aggression

Myth: *"They're doing it on purpose."*
Reality: Behavior changes are symptoms of brain changes, not personality.

As Alzheimer's progresses, several cognitive skills weaken:

Brain function lost	Behavior families see
Memory	Asking the same question repeatedly
Logic & reasoning	Arguments, suspicion, frustration
Language processing	Searching for words, misunderstanding
Spatial awareness	Getting lost or wandering
Impulse control	Anger outbursts, impatience

The brain cells responsible for **memory, judgment, and self-control** are physically deteriorating. When the person cannot express needs verbally, behavior becomes communication.

✅ **Behavior = Message.**
Anger may mean fear.
Repetition may mean anxiety.
Wandering may mean boredom, discomfort, or confusion.

When we stop asking **"Why are they acting like this?"** and instead ask **"What are they trying to tell me?"**, everything changes.

Common Behaviors and What They Really Mean

■1. Repeating the Same Questions

Example:
"Where are we going?"
"What time is it?"
"Did you see my keys?" *...five minutes later...*

Why it happens:
Short-term memory becomes weak. They may forget the answer moments after hearing it.

Hidden message:

- They are anxious or uncertain.
- They need reassurance, not information.

✅ **Pro Tip:**
Instead of repeating the answer with frustration, answer with comfort and calm tone.
If needed, write answers on a large visible board:

- "Today: Doctor at 3PM."
- "Dinner at 6PM."
  Visual cues reduce repetition dramatically.

■2. Arguments or Anger

The Alzheimer's brain struggles with:

- Confusion
- Feeling out of control
- Misunderstanding tone or words

Myth: *"They're just being stubborn."*
Truth: They are protecting themselves from a world that no longer makes sense.

✅ **Pro Tip:** You cannot win an argument with Alzheimer's. Trying will only create fear or aggression.

Use the **Three-Step De-escalation Strategy**:

1. **Validate feelings** ("I hear you're upset.")
2. **Stay calm** (speak softly, slow movements)
3. **Redirect attention** ("Let's sit and have tea.")

■3. Suspicion & Accusations

Example:

- "Someone stole my purse."
- "You're hiding things from me."
- "Strangers are in the house."

When memory fails, the brain fills in gaps with imagination. Losing objects or forgetting conversations leads to paranoia.

What not to say:
❌ "You're wrong."
❌ "No one would steal from you."
❌ "Stop being paranoid."

Even truthful corrections can feel like attacks.

✅ **Better response:**

- "Let's look for the purse together."
- "You're safe, and I'm here."

■4. Wandering

This is one of the most dangerous behaviors. Wandering happens because of:

- Restlessness
- Memory loss ("I need to go home" even when they're already home)
- Old habits (going to work, visiting family)
- Searching for someone

Safety Strategies:

- Put locks high or low on doors (not eye level)
- Use motion sensors or chimes
- Create a daily walking routine
- Provide meaningful activity so they don't roam out of boredom

■5. Nighttime Confusion & Sundowning

Many families report that evenings are the hardest time.

You may see:

- Agitation
- Pacing
- Restlessness
- Difficulty sleeping
- "I need to go now."

Why it happens:

- Light patterns upset the brain's internal clock
- Shadows cause fear or confusion
- Fatigue makes thinking harder

✅ How to Handle Arguments, Repetition, and Wandering with Calm Communication

1. Speak Like a Guide, Not a Corrector

Don't Say	Do Say
"You just asked me that five times!"	"We're having dinner soon. Would you like to help set the table?"
"That's not true."	"I can see why you'd feel that way. Let's check together."
"You're wrong."	"You're safe. I'm right here with you."

Tone matters more than words.

Rule: Alzheimer's will not remember what you said —but they will remember how you made them feel.

2. Use Simple, Clear Language

- One sentence at a time
- Use names instead of "he" or "she"
- Slow speech, softer voice
- Give one instruction, not many

Example:
❌ "Get dressed and come to the kitchen for breakfast."
✅ "Here is your shirt. Let's put it on first."

Small wins reduce stress.

3. Redirect Instead of Correcting

When someone is stuck on a thought:

✗ "Stop asking, I told you already."
✅ "Let's look at your photo album while we wait."

Activity changes focus without confrontation.

✅ Creating a Peaceful & Safe Home Environment

A calm environment reduces anger and confusion better than any argument.

✔ Lighting

- Bright daylight reduces shadows (shadows increase fear)
- Soft night lighting prevents confusion if they wake up

✔ Eliminate Noise Stress

- Turn off loud TV
- Avoid overlapping sounds (TV + music + conversation)
- Use calm music or nature sounds

✔ Remove Triggers

- Mirrors may confuse them ("Who is that stranger?")
- Clutter causes frustration
- Busy patterns on carpets can look like holes or water

✔ Predictable Routine = Predictable Feelings

The more the day repeats the same way, the safer the brain feels.

Real-Life Example: Reducing Nighttime Agitation

Family:
Samira cares for her father, who became restless every night. Around 8pm he paced, checked doors, and insisted "I need to go

home"—even though he *was* home. Nothing worked. He slept 3 hours a night, and Samira slept even less.

What was actually happening:

- Lights in the home were dim
- Shadows moved on walls and floors
- Routine changed every night
- No sleep schedule, no quiet wind-down

What the family tried:

✔ At 6pm, house lights were turned **brighter**, not dimmer
✔ TV turned off after dinner to reduce stimulation
✔ Soft music or Quran recitation played at night
✔ Short walk every afternoon
✔ Front door fitted with a quiet alarm
✔ Bedroom placed nightlight in hallway and bathroom

Results in 2 weeks:

✅ Nighttime pacing dropped
✅ He slept 6–7 hours
✅ He stopped trying to "go home"
✅ Samira got her sleep—and her sanity—back

The lesson: Evening agitation is rarely about anger.
It's about confusion, shadows, routines, and overstimulation.

Hidden Pitfalls Families Don't Realize

Even loving families accidentally make things worse:

❌ Explaining too much
❌ Asking "Don't you remember?"
❌ Speaking from another room
❌ Rushing or hurrying them
❌ Correcting details
❌ Using long sentences or multiple instructions

✅ The correct approach:

- Short
- Gentle
- Simple
- Patient
- Reassuring

Pro Tips to Calm Difficult Moments

✔ Give choices, not orders
"Would you like tea or juice?"

✔ Keep hands visible when speaking
Hidden hands feel threatening to the Alzheimer's brain

✔ Smile before speaking
The brain recognizes emotion faster than words

✔ Use touch gently
A hand on the shoulder can calm faster than a sentence

✔ Keep routines—for meals, baths, medications, bedtime
Routine reduces fear

One Sentence That Helps Almost Every Situation

"You're safe. I'm here with you."

It does not matter if the statement is repeated.
Repetition is comfort.

The Power of Environment Over Arguments

Families often try to fix behaviors with logic.
But Alzheimer's responds better to **environmental changes** than explanations.

Example changes that can stop anger:

- Add better lighting

- Reduce noise
- Keep walkways clear
- Provide familiar objects (favorite blanket, prayer beads, photos)
- Play calming music
- Create a bedtime ritual: warm drink, light talk, soft light

When the environment feels safe, behavior gets calmer.

In Summary

- Behavior is communication, not attitude
- You cannot win an argument with Alzheimer's
- Calm voice, gentle touch, and routine work better than logic
- A peaceful environment prevents problems before they start
- Nighttime agitation can be reduced with light, routine, and comfort

Families who learn these skills protect their loved one's dignity and reduce their own stress dramatically.

*Here is a clear, practical **Calming Communication Chart** perfect for caregivers to print or keep on the wall.*
*It shows **what to avoid, what to say instead**, and **why it works**.*

Calming Communication Chart for Alzheimer's Care

If the person says or does…	Avoid saying… (makes it worse)	Say this instead… (calms and redirects)	Why it works
Repeats the same question many times	"I already told you!" / "You're repeating yourself!"	"You're safe. We have an appointment at 3:00. Want to sit with me while we wait?"	Reassurance reduces anxiety; clear info + companionship stops the loop
Insists on going "home" (even if already home)	"You ARE home. Stop it."	"Tell me what you miss about home. Let's look at your photo album together."	Validates feelings and redirects attention without arguing
Accuses someone of stealing	"No one stole anything, you're imagining things!"	"Let's look for it together. I'm here to help."	Removes confrontation and builds safety
Gets angry or raises voice	"Calm down!" / "Stop yelling!"	Soft tone: "I'm here with you. Let's sit down and talk."	Soft voice triggers mirror calm; sitting feels safer
Refuses to bathe	"You HAVE to shower now!"	"Would you like a warm shower or a quick wash with warm towels?"	Offering choice gives control and reduces fear
Wandering or	"Sit down. You	"Let's take a	Redirects

If the person says or does…	Avoid saying… (makes it worse)	Say this instead… (calms and redirects)	Why it works
trying to leave	can't go anywhere."	little walk together inside. I could use the exercise."	movement instead of denying it
Confused about who you are	"How can you forget me?"	"I love spending time with you. I'm right here."	Emotion is more important than identity
Doesn't understand instructions	Long explanations	One simple step: "Here is your coat. Let's put it on together."	Too many words overwhelm; one step builds confidence
Cries or says "I want to go home"	"This is your home!"	"I know it's confusing. You're safe with me. Would you like tea?"	Comfort > correction; tea gives soothing distraction
Sundowning / evening agitation	"Stop pacing. Go to sleep."	"Let's sit with some music and a warm drink."	Calm routine signals the brain to relax
Confused by mirrors	"It's just you!"	Remove or cover mirror	Environment change works faster than explanation
Won't eat	"You have to eat or you'll get sick."	"Try one bite. It smells good. Want to eat together?"	Social eating increases appetite and reduces pressure

Bonus Communication Rules

Rule	Why it matters
Use a calm, slow voice	Alzheimer's brain processes tone before words

Rule	Why it matters
Approach from the front, not behind	Prevents startle and fear
Smile before speaking	Facial emotion calms the nervous system
Use touch gently	A hand on the shoulder builds connection
Give 1 instruction at a time	Multi-step directions create confusion

✅**Quick Script Starters You Can Use Anytime:**

- **"You're safe. I'm here with you."**
- **"Let's do this together."**
- **"I can see you're upset. How about we sit for a bit?"**
- **"That sounds important. Tell me more."**

These phrases soothe fear and protect dignity.

CHAPTER 4: Caring at Home – Daily Routines & Safety

Building Structure, Comfort, and Security for Alzheimer's Care

Home can be the safest and most loving place for a person with Alzheimer's—**if the environment supports their changing abilities.**
This chapter shows how to build daily routines, prevent accidents, manage bathing and medication, handle sundowning, and create a home that protects dignity without taking away independence.

✅ *Why Daily Routine Matters*

A routine is not just organization—it is **medicine for the Alzheimer's brain.**

Lack of routine causes:

- Anxiety
- Repetition
- Wandering
- Nighttime confusion
- Agitation

When the day is predictable, **the brain relaxes**.

✅The "Same-Time Rule"

If meals, bathing, medication, and sleep happen at the **same time every day**, behavior problems decrease.

Example daily flow:

- Wake up → Wash → Breakfast → Light activity

- Afternoon rest → Snack → Music/walk
- Evening routine → Soft lighting → Bedtime

The brain cannot keep memories—but it can remember patterns.

✅ Home Safety Checklist

A safe home prevents falls, wandering, burns, medication mistakes, and nighttime injuries.

✅ General Safety

✔ Remove loose rugs
✔ Clear walking paths
✔ Bright lighting (bulbs 2–3x brighter than average home)
✔ Lock up cleaning products, tools, knives
✔ Keep emergency contacts visible on the fridge
✔ Use nightlights in hallway, bathroom, and bedroom
✔ Avoid glass tables, sharp corners, clutter

✅ Medication Safety

✔ Store medications in a locked cabinet
✔ Use a weekly pill organizer
✔ One person should manage medications—**not shared responsibility**
✔ Keep a written medication list on the fridge for emergencies

✅ Wandering Prevention

✔ Install door chimes or alarms
✔ Add locks high or low on doors (not eye level)
✔ Place "STOP" or curtain over exit doors
✔ Provide daily physical activity—exercise reduces wandering

Safety Fact:
Most wandering happens between **6pm and midnight**,

especially during sundowning.

✅Bathing, Dressing, Cooking, Medication: Step-by-Step Solutions

✅Bathing

Bathing is stressful for many families. Alzheimer's may cause:

- Fear of falling
- Embarrassment
- Confusion about water
- Feeling cold

✅How to make bathing calm

✔ Warm the bathroom first
✔ Lay out everything before starting
✔ Use soft voice and step-by-step instructions
✔ Offer choices: "Shower or warm towel bath?"
✔ Use non-slip mats and handheld showerhead
✔ Never rush—slow movements equal safety

✅What NOT to do

❌Don't argue
❌Don't surprise them by turning on water suddenly
❌Don't close doors aggressively—trapped feeling increases panic

Pro-Tip:
If bathing becomes impossible, use **towel baths** or **bath wipes** temporarily. Cleanliness matters—**but safety matters more.**

✅Dressing

People with Alzheimer's may forget the order of clothing or

wear layers incorrectly.

✅ **Solutions**

✔ Lay out outfits in order: underwear → shirt → pants → socks
✔ Remove extra clothing from closet to avoid confusion
✔ Choose soft, easy-to-pull clothing
✔ Avoid small buttons or tricky zippers

Encourage independence:
Give one task: "Put your arms through these sleeves."
Too many instructions = frustration.

✅ **Cooking & Meals**

Cooking can be dangerous if memory loss is advanced.

✅ **Safety rules**

✔ Remove or unplug stove knobs if needed
✔ Use microwave instead of stove
✔ Keep knives out of sight
✔ Install smoke alarms
✔ Never leave them alone in the kitchen while cooking

Mealtime Behavior Tips
✔ Small meals more often
✔ Eat together—social eating increases appetite
✔ Avoid arguing about food
✔ Use plates with contrast color (white plate on dark table)

✅ **Medication Management**

One of the leading causes of hospitalization in Alzheimer's patients is **medication errors.**

✅ Assign ONE caregiver as medication manager
✅ Use pill organizers with labels
✅ Set alarms for dose times

✅Keep water nearby to prevent choking
✅Keep a written log

✅**Sleep and Sundowning Problems**

Evening hours are often the hardest. The brain becomes more confused when:

- Light changes
- Shadows appear
- The day's fatigue builds
- Noise from TV or visitors overwhelms them

✅**How to reduce sundowning**

✔ Increase light in the house from late afternoon
✔ Quiet environment after dinner
✔ Warm drink (milk, tea, herbal)
✔ Soothing music or prayer/recitation
✔ No caffeine after 3pm
✔ Short walk in the afternoon
✔ Remove mirrors at night—reflections can cause fear

✅**What to say when they want to "go home"**

❌ "You ARE home!"
✅"Tell me about the house you miss. Let's look at photos together."

Emotional truth matters more than factual truth.

✅**Managing Accidents, Hallucinations & Difficult Moments**

✅**Accidents (urine, stool, spills)**

Do not shame. Do not show frustration.

✅Calmly say:

"It's okay. Let's get cleaned up."

Use easy-to-remove clothing
Use waterproof mattress covers
Keep spare clothes ready
Take bathroom breaks on schedule

✅ Hallucinations

They may see animals, strangers, or shapes that aren't real.

Do NOT say:
❌ "That's not real! Stop imagining things!"
This increases fear and distrust.

Do say:
✅ "I know that looks scary. You're safe. I'm here."
✅ "Let's go sit in the other room where it feels comfortable."

If hallucinations are frequent, talk to their doctor—sometimes lighting, dehydration, or medication can cause them.

ROOM-BY-ROOM SAFETY GUIDE

✅ Bedroom

✔ Nightlight
✔ Bed rails if needed
✔ Clear path to bathroom
✔ Soft carpet or no carpet
✔ Extra blanket visible and easy to reach

✅ Bathroom

✔ Non-slip mats
✔ Grab bars in shower and near toilet
✔ Handheld showerhead
✔ Warm room (cold causes resistance)
✔ Lock removed or replaced with privacy latch

✅ **Kitchen**

✔ Knives and scissors hidden
✔ Stove knobs removed if they wander
✔ Fire extinguisher visible
✔ Cleaning chemicals locked

✅ **Living Room**

✔ No glass tables
✔ Remove clutter
✔ Soft lighting
✔ TV not too loud (loud noise triggers agitation)

✅ **Front Door**

✔ Chimes or alarms
✔ Deadbolt above or below eye level
✔ Curtains or film to reduce desire to "go outside"

✅ **Outdoor**

✔ Secure gate
✔ Remove slippery surfaces
✔ Hide car keys
✔ Consider ID bracelet with contact information

Printable Daily Care Schedule

(You can print or adapt this exactly.)

Time	Activity	Goal
7:00 AM	Wake up, bathroom, wash face	Gentle start to day
7:30 AM	Breakfast + medication	Calm, structured routine
8:00–10:00 AM	Light activity (walk, music, simple chores)	Reduce restlessness, wandering

Time	Activity	Goal
10:30 AM	Snack + hydration	Prevent dehydration agitation
11:00–12:00 PM	Quiet activity (puzzles, photos, prayer)	Mental stimulation
12:30 PM	Lunch	Balanced meal
1:30–2:30 PM	Rest / nap	Prevent evening agitation
3:00 PM	Outdoor or indoor light exercise	Improve sleep
4:00 PM	Snack + calming music	Transition into evening
5:30 PM	Dinner	Predictable mealtime
6:30 PM	Soft light, TV off, quiet routine	Reduce sundowning
8:00 PM	Bath & pajamas	Wind-down ritual
9:00 PM	Bedtime with nightlight	Safety + comfort

Routine protects the caregiver and the loved one.

✅ Real Family Example

Nadia cared for her mother who became restless every evening — pacing, asking to leave, loudly calling for her husband who had passed away years earlier.

Mistakes they didn't realize:

- Lights were low
- No evening routine
- TV was loud
- Too much stimulation

What they changed:
✔ Bright lights turned on at 5pm
✔ Family dinner at same time

✔ Soft music afterward
✔ TV kept off
✔ Warm shower before bed
✔ Nightlight in hallway and bathroom

Result:
Within 10 days, agitation dropped, pacing stopped, and her mother began sleeping 6+ hours a night.

✅ **Final Takeaways**

- Alzheimer's behavior improves with routine
- Home must be simple, safe, calm
- Safety changes prevent emergencies
- Small adjustments reduce arguments, falls, and nighttime confusion
- Dignity and independence are still possible—with support

CHAPTER 5: The Role of the Family Caregiver: Why Love Is Not Enough

If you are reading this chapter, you have likely become something you never trained to be: a family caregiver. This role is not chosen; it is bestowed by circumstance, a seismic shift in your identity and life's trajectory. We often enter this role armed with one powerful, yet insufficient, tool: love. This chapter will move beyond the platitudes to explore the brutal, beautiful, and counterintuitive truths of caregiving. We will expose the silent epidemic of caregiver burnout, not as a personal failure, but as a systemic collapse of support. We will dismantle the "solutions" that backfire and illuminate the path to sustainable care—a path that requires strategy, delegation, and, most critically, self-preservation.

The Superstar Myth: What Caregivers Really Do (And Why It's More Than "Helping")

The Common Misconception: The public imagines caregiving as a mix of gentle companionship and simple chores—cooking meals, offering an arm to lean on. It's seen as an extension of a good relationship, a "payback" for a lifetime of love.

The Interesting Angle/The Reality: Family caregiving is a high-stakes, multi-skilled profession performed by amateurs in a state of perpetual crisis. Your real job description is one of the most complex in the world, encompassing roles you are likely unprepared for:

•**The Project Manager:** You are no longer just scheduling a doctor's appointment. You are managing a complex web of medical professionals, insurance claims, medication schedules, and legal paperwork. A single error—a missed dose, a mis-filed claim—can have catastrophic consequences.

•**The EMT & Risk Assessor:** Your home must be transformed into a secure facility. You are constantly scanning for fall hazards, assessing wandering risks, and managing choking dangers. You are the first responder to crises, from a sudden fall to a violent outburst, often with no training.

•**The Behavioral Detective:** The person you love may say things they don't mean and act in ways you don't recognize. Your job is to decode the unmet need behind the aggression. Is the sundowning agitation due to hunger, pain, or a simple change in barometric pressure? You are solving puzzles with missing pieces every single day.

•**The Keeper of the Flame:** You become the guardian of your loved one's personhood. You are the one who tells the stories they've forgotten, who affirms their values, and who sees the person beyond the disease. This is emotionally sacred and profoundly draining work.

Pro-Tip: Reframe your role from "caregiver" to "care manager." Your primary job is not to personally execute every task, but to orchestrate the care. This mental shift is the first step toward preventing burnout and building a sustainable system.

Hidden Pitfall: The Competence Trap. The better you become at managing everything, the more invisible your labor becomes, and the less others feel compelled to help. You create a system of dependency where you are the sole, irreplaceable component, guaranteeing your own eventual collapse.

The Triad of Burnout: Stress, Guilt, and the Exhaustion That Sleep Can't Fix

The emotional toll of caregiving is well-documented, but its depths are often misunderstood. It's not just about being tired; it's about a fundamental erosion of the self.

1. Chronic Stress: The Body Keeps the Score

This isn't ordinary stress. It's the toxic, relentless strain of hyper-vigilance. Your nervous system is permanently set to "high alert," listening for a fall in the night, anticipating the next crisis. This state floods your body with cortisol, leading to physical symptoms: insomnia, weight changes, a weakened immune system (you're always getting sick), and a higher risk for chronic conditions like hypertension and heart disease. You are literally making yourself sick to care for someone else.

2. Ambiguous Loss: The Source of the Pain

The concept of **Ambiguous Loss**, developed by Dr. Pauline Boss, is the critical key to understanding caregiver grief. Your loved one is **physically present but psychologically absent**. This is a unique and torturous form of grief. There is no closure, no clear line to cross. You are grieving a living person. Society doesn't recognize your loss, so you are often left to mourn in silence, which fuels a deep, isolating sadness beneath the surface of your daily tasks.

3. The Guilt That Never Sleeps

Caregiver guilt is a predatory emotion. It feeds on your most vulnerable moments.

•**Role Reversal Guilt:** The discomfort of parenting your parent.

•**Self-Care Guilt:** The feeling that taking an hour for yourself is stealing it from your loved one.
•** Anger Guilt:** The shame of feeling resentful or losing your temper with someone who is sick.
•**Grief Guilt:** The secret wish for it all to be over, followed by immediate self-loathing.

Pro-Tip: Name Your Guilt. When you feel guilt, speak its full name: "This is my self-care guilt because I booked a massage." "This is my anger guilt because I yelled when she spilled her medicine." Naming it robs it of its amorphous power and allows you to challenge its validity.

Hidden Pitfall: The Martyrdom Trap. Society often glorifies the self-sacrificing caregiver. This narrative is dangerous. It makes you believe that suffering is a measure of your love. In reality, martyrdom leads to resentment, poorer care, and ultimately, abandonment of the role when you break down completely.

Flawed Solutions: Why Common "Fixes" Backfire

When caregivers reach their breaking point, they often grasp for logical solutions. Unfortunately, many of these intuitive strategies are fundamentally flawed.

Flawed Solution #1: “I Just Need to Try Harder.”

•**The Logic:** If I’m overwhelmed, I must not be efficient or dedicated enough. The solution is to work longer hours, sleep less, and eliminate my own needs.
•**Why It Fails:** Caregiving is a bottomless pit. There is always more to do. The problem is not your effort but the volume of the

demand. "Trying harder" is like trying to bail out a flooding boat with a teaspoon instead of plugging the leak. It accelerates burnout without addressing the core issue: you need more hands on deck, not more hustle.

Flawed Solution #2: "My Family Will Step Up."

•**The Logic:** I'll call a family meeting, explain the situation, and everyone will naturally divide the responsibilities.
•**Why It Fails:** This assumes a level of shared commitment, skill, and availability that rarely exists. Sibling dynamics, geographic distance, and denial about the severity of the illness often sabotage this plan. The primary caregiver, usually one person, ends up delegating not tasks, but the anxiety about the tasks, and then often re-doing the work because it wasn't done "correctly." This leads to the "designated martyr" phenomenon.

Flawed Solution #3: "I Can Handle This Alone to Protect My Loved One."

•**The Logic:** Introducing outside help (a home health aide, respite care) will confuse, agitate, or embarrass my loved one. I know them best, so I should be the only one providing care.
•**Why It Fails:** This is perhaps the most tragic and common pitfall. While meant as protection, it is a form of isolation that harms both the caregiver and the care recipient. The person with dementia may actually benefit from a new, patient face without the complex emotional history. More importantly, by refusing to introduce help, you are creating a fragile, single-point-of-failure system. When you inevitably get sick or burn out, the transition for your loved one will be far more traumatic than a gradual, managed introduction of help.

Do These Solutions Work? They solve the immediate problem of feeling proactive, but they are tactical fixes for a strategic problem. They provide a temporary illusion of control while systematically ensuring a larger collapse down the road.

Knowing When You Need Help: The Inevitability of a Team

The question is not if you will need help, but when. The best time to build your lifeboat is before the ship starts taking on water. You need to act when you notice the following:

•**The Health Barometer:** Your own health is declining—chronic pain, persistent colds, new or worsening conditions.
•**The Patience Gauge:** You are irritable, snapping at your loved one, your children, or coworkers over minor inconveniences.
•**The Joy Index:** You have abandoned hobbies and social connections and can't remember the last time you felt genuine laughter or lightheartedness.
•**The Resentment Monitor:** You feel deep resentment toward your loved one, your siblings, or the world in general. This is a major red flag that the balance between duty and self has been completely lost.

Finding Support Services: Building Your Care Coalition

Shifting from a solo act to a conductor requires building a formal and informal coalition.

1. Formal Support: The Professional Corps

•**Respite Care:** This is not a luxury; it is a medical necessity for the caregiver. It is scheduled, non-negotiable time off. **Pro-Tip:** Start with short, positive exposures. Don't introduce a respite worker for a full day. Have them come for two hours to

"help Mom with her crossword puzzle" while you "run a quick errand."
•**Geriatric Care Manager (GCM):** A GCM is a paid professional, often a social worker or nurse, who acts as your expert guide. They can assess needs, find resources, and even be a neutral, professional voice in family conflicts. They are worth their weight in gold for their expertise and objectivity.
•**Support Groups (In-Person or Online):** The magic of a support group isn't in the advice; it's in the validation. Hearing others articulate your exact feelings is profoundly healing. It dismantles the isolation and proves you are not going crazy.

2. Informal Support: The "Care Convoy"
Stop waiting for people to offer help. Most people want to help but are paralyzed by not knowing what to do.

•**The Specific Ask:** Instead of "Let me know if you need anything," train people to respond to direct, time-bound requests. Create a shared online calendar (like Google Calendar or Lotsa Helping Hands) with specific tasks: "Bring a meal on Tuesday," "Sit with Dad from 1-3 pm on Thursday," "Mow the lawn this weekend."
•**Delegate by Affinity:** The sibling who is bad with hands-on care might be excellent at managing finances. The friend who is uncomfortable with medical tasks can be tasked with walking the dog or picking up groceries.

Case Study: The Architect of Her Own Burnout

Subject: Michael, 58, a retired project manager caring for his wife, Sarah, with early-onset Alzheimer's.

The Flawed Strategy: Michael approached caregiving like his last major project. He created intricate spreadsheets for medications, a color-coded calendar for appointments, and a flawless daily routine. He was the CEO, CFO, and sole employee of "Sarah's Care, Inc." He refused his children's offers to help, saying, "I've got a system. It's easier if I just do it." He was solving for efficiency, not for sustainability.

The Cracks Appear: Michael's system was technically perfect, but it was brittle. When Sarah's sleep patterns reversed, his schedule shattered. He was up all night, surviving on caffeine and willpower. His children saw his exhaustion but were locked out of his system. His identity became solely "Sarah's caregiver," and the competent, funny man they knew vanished.

The Breaking Point: Michael developed crippling back pain from assisting Sarah. His own doctor told him he needed rest and physical therapy. The terror Michael felt was not for his own health, but for his system: "If I go down, who will run the spreadsheet? Who knows her routine?" His perfect system had no backup plan.

The Pivot: In a moment of desperation, Michael's daughter didn't ask to help; she insisted on being trained. She sat with him for a weekend, not as a helper, but as an apprentice. She learned the "system." She then used her skills to modify it, creating simplified, laminated checklists and setting up automated pill dispensers. She brought in a respite worker twice a week, not to replace Michael, but to become a familiar, trained part of the system.

The Lesson: Michael learned that the ultimate project management skill is delegation and redundancy. "My love for Sarah was what started this," he said, "but it was my ego that nearly destroyed it. Letting go of control wasn't a failure of love; it was the only way to ensure her care would continue, even if I couldn't be the one to provide every minute of it."

The journey of the family caregiver is a marathon run at a sprint pace, with no finish line in sight. The central, counterintuitive truth you must embrace is this: **The single most important person to care for in this journey is yourself.** Your well-being is the foundation upon which everything else rests. To care for another with grace and endurance, you must tend to your own health, your own spirit, and your own life with the same fierce dedication you offer them. Love is the fuel, but strategy, support, and self-compassion are the map and the spare tires. Do not let your love become the reason you both falter. Build your coalition, share the burden, and grant yourself the permission to be both a devoted caregiver and a whole, human being.

CHAPTER 6: Helping Children & Teenagers Understand: Beyond "Be Nice to Grandma"

When dementia enters a family, a silent seismic shift occurs, and the youngest members are often standing on the most unstable ground. For a child or teenager, the gradual disappearance of a beloved grandparent is a unique form of loss—one without a clear explanation or the rituals of a funeral. They are left with a confusing presence where a person used to be. This chapter moves beyond simplistic advice to provide a strategic, evidence-based guide for helping young people navigate this painful journey. We will dismantle common myths, explore the data on their emotional worlds, and provide a blueprint for fostering resilient, adaptive relationships that can survive the ravages of memory loss.

The Unseen Impact: Data on the Youngest Caregivers and Grievers

The common misconception is that children are resilient and largely unaffected by a grandparent's dementia. The reality, revealed by the data, is that they are deeply impacted, often in ways they lack the vocabulary to express.

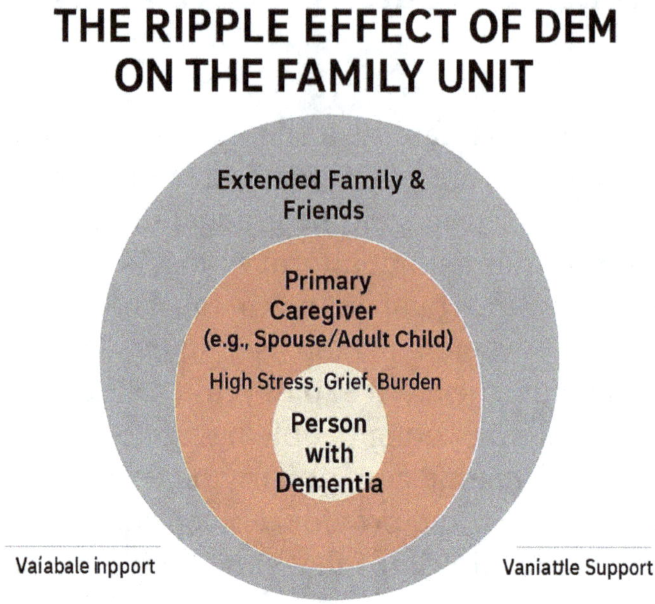

Figure 1: The Ripple Effect of Dementia on the Family Unit

[Conceptual Diagram: A series of concentric circles.]
Center Circle: "Person with Dementia"
Second Circle: "Primary Caregiver (e.g., Spouse/Adult Child)" - Label: "High Stress, Grief, Burden"
Third Circle: "Children & Teenagers in the Home" - Label: "The Secondary Patients: Experiencing significant anxiety, behavioral changes, and role shifts."
Outer Circle: "Extended Family & Friends" - Label: "Variable Support"

Caption: Dementia's impact radiates outward, directly affecting the emotional and psychological well-being of children and teenagers in the household, who often become "secondary patients."

Consider the following research findings:

•**Prevalence:** A study published in the Journal of Alzheimer's Disease found that over **10% of children** live in a household where they are exposed to a family member with dementia, indicating this is a widespread childhood experience.
•**Emotional Toll:** Research from the American Academy of Child and Adolescent Psychiatry shows that children in these situations report significantly higher levels of **anxiety, embarrassment, and social withdrawal** than their peers. A UK study found that **44% of young carers** (many supporting someone with dementia) reported mental health problems.
•**The Knowledge Gap:** A survey by Alzheimer's Research UK revealed a critical insight: **Nearly 60% of adults** believe that a lack of understanding about dementia among the public is a major barrier to support. This gap is even wider for children, who are rarely given an honest, age-appropriate explanation.

The Interesting Angle/The Fact People Get Wrong:

The Myth: "We don't want to scare the children, so we'll just say Grandma is getting old and forgetful."

The Reality: Silence and euphemisms are more frightening than the truth. A child's brain is a meaning-making machine. When adults are visibly stressed, a loved one acts erratically, and no one provides a coherent explanation, children will invent their own. These explanations are often rooted in self-blame ("I must have done something wrong") or catastrophic thinking ("Everyone I love will disappear like this"). Providing a clear, medical framework for the changes is an act of reassurance, not of fear-mongering.

Explaining the Invisible: The "Broken Computer in Grandpa's Head"

The Common (Flawed) Solutions & Why They Fail:

1.**The "Nothing's Wrong" Approach:** Hiding the diagnosis and pretending everything is normal.

•**Why It Fails:** It invalidates the child's own observations and instincts. They know something is wrong. When their reality is denied, they learn not to trust their own senses or the adults around them, leading to anxiety and insecurity.

2.**The "Just Be Nice" Mandate:** Instructing a child to be patient and kind without context.

•**Why It Fails:** This places an unfair emotional burden on the child. It's like asking someone to fix a broken leg with a kind word. Without tools or understanding, the child is set up for failure, leading to frustration and guilt when they inevitably can't manage the loved one's behavior.

3.**The Forced Interaction:** Insisting on visits or lengthy contact despite a child's clear discomfort.

•**Why It Fails:** This transforms a relationship based on love into a stressful obligation. It associates the loved one with feelings of fear and pressure, potentially damaging the bond permanently.

The Pro-Tip Solution: Use a Concrete, Mechanical Analogy.

The most effective way to explain Alzheimer's to a child is to compare the brain to a familiar, complex machine—a computer.

The Script (Ages 5-12):
"Your grandpa's brain is like a supercomputer that controls everything he thinks, remembers, and feels. Lately, a sickness called Alzheimer's has been causing some wires to get crossed

and some files to get lost. That's why he sometimes can't find the file with your name in it, even though he loves you very much. It's why the computer might glitch and make him say or do things that seem confusing or scary. It's not Grandpa being mean; it's the sickness messing with his computer. We can't fix the computer, but we can learn to be good, patient tech supporters."

For Teenagers, you can be more specific, mentioning plaques and tangles as "corrupted files" or "viruses" that disrupt communication between the brain's hardware.

Hidden Pitfall: Avoid Blaming Age. Do not say, "Grandma is just old." This creates a fear of aging and can lead to negative stereotypes about all older people. It also minimizes a specific disease into a universal inevitability.

Navigating the Emotional Storm: From Embarrassment to Empathy

Children and teens express their complex grief differently. Recognizing these behaviors as symptoms of underlying distress is the first step toward helping.

Table 1: Decoding Emotional Reactions & Strategic Responses

Emotional Reaction	Common Behavioral Signs	What's Really Happening	Strategic Adult Response
Fear & Anxiety	Clinginess, nightmares, fear of the loved one, somatic complaints (stomach aches).	Fear of the unknown, worry that they or their parents will "catch" the disease, feeling unsafe.	**Reassure & Demystify:** "This disease isn't contagious. Your brain is healthy. We are safe." Maintain firm routines to create stability.
Embarrassment (Teens)	Avoiding visits, reluctance to be seen in public with the loved one, withdrawal.	A developmentally normal desire to fit in, clashing with a grandparent's "abnormal" behavior.	**Validate & Reframe:** "It's okay to feel embarrassed. That's normal. Imagine how he must feel, losing control in public."
Anger & Resentment	Acting out, anger toward parents or the loved one, irritability.	Anger at the situation, grief over lost attention, frustration that	**Normalize & Ventilate:** "It's completely fair to be angry that this is happening. I get

Emotional Reaction	Common Behavioral Signs	What's Really Happening	Strategic Adult Response
		family life has changed.	angry too. It's not fair. Let's go shoot some hoops and talk about it."
Guilt	Trying to be "perfect," asking "Was it something I did?", withdrawing.	Magical thinking: the child believes their actions caused the disease or can cure it.	**Be Explicit & Absolve:** "Listen to me: Nothing you ever did, said, or thought caused this. This is a disease, and it is no one's fault."
Withdrawal	Loss of interest in the loved one, preferring screen time, silence.	Emotional self-protection. The pain of the "new" relationship is too great, so they disengage.	**Offer Low-Pressure Connection:** "You don't have to talk. Want to just sit and watch his favorite old movie with us for 15 minutes? No pressure."

Pro-Tip: Separate the Person from the Disease. Consistently label challenging behaviors as "the Alzheimer's talking." This helps the child mentally file the distressing event under "sickness" rather than "Grandma doesn't love me anymore," preserving the internal image of their loving grandparent.

Involving Them Safely: The "Micro-Task" Methodology

The goal is not to make children into miniature caregivers but to empower them as "contributors." The key is assigning micro-tasks—small, manageable, and age-appropriate activities that provide a sense of agency without burden.

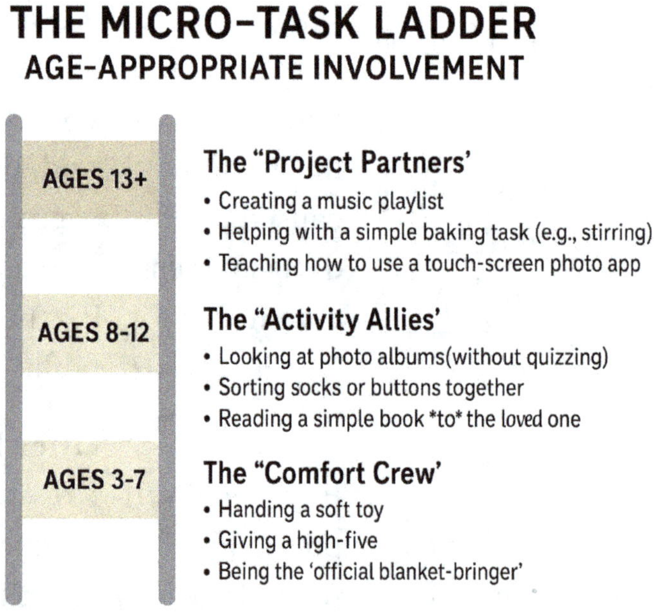

Figure 2: The Micro-Task Ladder: Age-Appropriate Involvement

RUNG 1: AGES 3-7
- Title: The "Comfort Crew"
- Tasks: Handing a soft toy, giving a high-five, being the "official blanket-bringer," pressing play on a music box.

RUNG 2: AGES 8-12

- Title: The "Activity Allies"
- Tasks: Looking at photo albums (without quizzing), sorting socks or buttons together, reading a simple book *to* the loved one.

RUNG 3: AGES 13+
- Title: The "Project Partners"
- Tasks: Creating a music playlist, helping with a simple baking task (e.g., stirring), teaching how to use a touch-screen photo app.

Caption: Involvement should be a choice, not a chore. This ladder provides a framework for meaningful, safe, and developmentally appropriate ways for young people to connect.

Hidden Pitfall: Parentification. Never confide in a child as a peer. Do not share your financial worries, your exhaustion, or your frustrations with other family members. This reverses the parent-child roles, forcing the child to bear an emotional weight that can crush their own development. Your child is your child, not your co-therapist.

Connection Beyond Words: Activities That Soothe the Amygdala

As language centers deteriorate in the brain, the emotional core (the limbic system, including the amygdala) remains largely intact. The most successful activities bypass cognition and speak directly to the senses and emotions.

The Most Common Flawed Activity: The Memory Test.

•**What it is:** Holding up a photo and asking, "Do you remember who this is?"

•**Why it Fails:** It highlights their disability, causing shame, anxiety, and agitation. It focuses on what is lost, rather than what remains.

Pro-Tip Solutions: Focus on the "Feeling Brain."

1. **Music Therapy:** Create a playlist of music from the loved one's late teens and early twenties (ages 15-25). This music is emotionally hardwired and can trigger positive memories and calmness, even in late stages. Don't ask if they remember it; just listen together.
2. **Sensory Kits:** Assemble a box with various textures: soft velvet, smooth worry stones, a bristly hairbrush, a cool metal spoon. Sensory stimulation can be calming and engaging without the need for conversation.
3. **Simple, Purposeful Tasks:** Folding laundry (washcloths are easy), wiping a table, or gardening (planting a bulb, watering). These activities provide a sense of normalcy and purpose.
4. **Animal-Assisted Interaction:** If possible, the presence of a calm, trained therapy dog can reduce anxiety and provide a non-judgmental point of connection for both the child and the loved one.

Case Study: Sofia's Story - From Fear to Friendship

The Struggle: Sofia, a bright and sensitive 9-year-old, had always shared a special bond with her Abuela Maria, who taught her to bake and spoke to her in Spanish. When Maria was diagnosed with Alzheimer's, the changes were subtle at first. She'd forget a word, repeat a story. Then, during a visit, Maria became suddenly agitated, accusing Sofia of stealing her favorite scarf. She shouted in a mix of Spanish and English, her face contorted in anger. Sofia, terrified, hid in her room for the rest of the visit. After that, she refused to see Abuela, claiming she was "busy with homework." Her parents, stressed and grieving themselves, alternated between pleading ("But she's your Abuela!") and scolding ("You're being selfish!"), which only deepened Sofia's withdrawal and guilt.

The Flawed Solutions in Action: The "Just Be Nice" mandate and "Forced Interaction" were failing spectacularly. Sofia was not selfish; she was traumatized and lacked the framework to understand the sudden, frightening change in her beloved grandmother.

The Turning Point: Sofia's mother, realizing their approach was breaking the family further, decided to try a new strategy. She sat with Sofia and used the "broken computer" analogy. Sofia listened intently, her eyes widening. "So... Abuela's brain is just glitching?" she asked. "It's not that she doesn't love me?" The relief was palpable.

Next, her mother retired the stressful, expectation-filled baking sessions. She introduced a new, failure-proof micro-task. She gave Sofia a "job": to be Abuela's "Chief Hand-Holder and Music DJ." Their next visit was structured and short (20 minutes). Sofia didn't have to talk. She simply held her Abuela's hand and played a playlist of old Mexican boleros. At first, Maria was withdrawn. But as a familiar song filled the room, she began to hum. Then, she squeezed Sofia's hand. She didn't say Sofia's name, but she looked at her, and for a moment, the fear was gone from her eyes. They sat, hand-in-hand, listening to the music.

The Resolution: Sofia didn't magically become unafraid overnight, but she now had a role and an explanation. The visits became brief sensory sessions—brushing Abuela's hair, sharing a smoothie, listening to music. The pressure for a "normal"

conversation was gone. Sofia learned that while she had lost the Abuela who taught her recipes, she could still be a compassionate friend to the Abuela she had now. She moved from a place of fear to a place of empathy, all because the adults in her life replaced pressure with tools and understanding.
Helping a child navigate a loved one's dementia is one of the most challenging tasks a family can face. It requires us to abandon simplistic scripts and lean into complex, emotionally intelligent strategies. By replacing silence with clear analogies, validating difficult emotions, and facilitating connection through micro-tasks and sensory activities, we do more than just manage a crisis. We teach our children a masterclass in empathy, resilience, and the enduring nature of love—a love that is not contingent on memory or cognitive ability, but on the courageous choice to show up, again and again, with compassion and understanding. In doing so, we honor the relationship that was, and we build a new, meaningful one that can endure to the very end.

CHAPTER 7: Money, Legal Planning & Future Decisions: The Logistics of Love

The journey through Alzheimer's and other dementias is not just a medical or emotional one; it is a profound financial and legal undertaking. While love may be the foundation of care, it is a solid legal and financial plan that builds the walls of security and stability. This chapter moves beyond the intimidating jargon to provide a clear-eyed, practical guide to the logistics of care. We will expose the staggering, often-hidden costs, demystify the critical legal documents, and provide a strategic framework for making unified family decisions before a crisis strips away your options. The most compassionate act you can perform for your loved one—and for yourself—is to plan for the storm while the sun is still shining.

The Staggering Cost of Care: Navigating a Financial Minefield

The common misconception is that Medicare or standard health insurance will cover the long-term care required for dementia. This is one of the most costly and devastating assumptions a family can make.

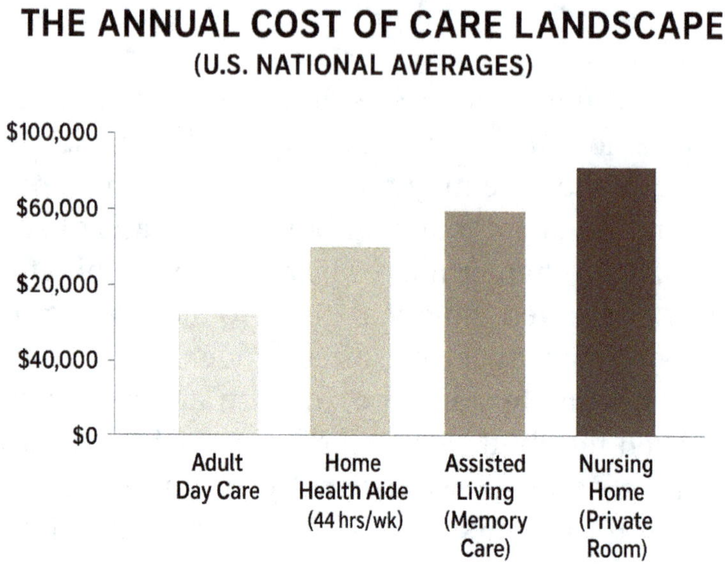

Figure 1: The Annual Cost of Care Landscape (U.S. National Averages)

[A bar chart comparing the annual cost of different types of care.]

- Adult Day Care: _______________~$20,000
- Home Health Aide (44 hrs/wk): ________~$60,000
- Assisted Living (Memory Care): ________~$72,000
- Nursing Home (Private Room): _________~$108,000

Caption: Based on data from Genworth's 2023 Cost of Care Survey. These are national median figures; costs can be 50-100% higher in major metropolitan areas. Memory care often carries a 20-30% premium over standard assisted living.

The Interesting Angle/The Fact People Get Wrong:

The Myth: "We'll cross that bridge when we come to it. For now, we can manage at home."

The Reality: The "bridge" is already on fire, and the cost of care is a five-alarm blaze. Dementia is a marathon, not a sprint, and the cumulative costs over 5-10 years can effortlessly decimate a lifetime of savings. The average out-of-pocket cost for a family caring for someone with dementia is nearly **$10,000 per year**, and that's before considering paid care facilities.

Breaking Down the Costs:

•**Home Care:** The most variable cost. It includes:

•**Home Modifications:** Grab bars, ramps, wheelchair-accessible showers ($1,500 - $10,000+).
•**Safety Technology:** Monitoring systems, GPS trackers ($50 - $150/month).
•**Paid Help:** The biggest expense. A home health aide for 44 hours a week averages **$60,000 annually**. 24/7 care can exceed $200,000 per year.
•**Memory Care / Assisted Living:** A all-inclusive monthly fee covering housing, meals, and specialized care. The national median is **$6,000 per month**, but can easily reach $8,000-$10,000 in high-cost areas.
•**Nursing Home Care:** The most expensive option, for when medical needs are too high for memory care. A private room averages **$9,000 per month** or $108,000 annually.

Pro-Tip: Activate All Available Resources Immediately. Don't wait until savings are depleted.

•**Veterans Benefits:** The VA Aid and Attendance pension can provide significant monthly funds for wartime veterans or their surviving spouses.

•**Long-Term Care Insurance:** If your loved one has a policy, understand the triggers for benefits (often requiring help with 2+ Activities of Daily Living) and file the claim as soon as they are eligible.
•**Medicaid:** This is the primary payer for long-term care in the U.S., but only for those who have exhausted nearly all their assets. The rules are complex and vary by state. **Consult an Elder Law Attorney early** to understand the "spend-down" rules and potential asset protection strategies, which must be implemented years in advance.

Hidden Pitfall: The Hidden Cost of the Family Caregiver. The financial impact isn't just out-of-pocket expenses. A 2021 AARP report valued the unpaid care provided by family caregivers at **$600 billion annually**. This often comes in the form of reduced hours, leaving the workforce, or lost career advancement opportunities for the caregiver, impacting their own future Social Security benefits and retirement savings.

Power of Attorney & Advanced Planning: The Legal Cornerstones of Care

Without the proper legal documents, you have no legal authority to manage your loved one's finances or make healthcare decisions on their behalf. Once they lose mental capacity, it is too late.

The Common (Flawed) Solution: "My name is on their bank account, so I'm fine." or "I'm the spouse, I can make all the decisions."

Why It Fails: A joint bank account exposes your assets to your loved one's creditors and can create gift tax complications.

Simply being a spouse does not give you automatic authority to sell their property or make certain medical choices if they are incapacitated. Without specific legal documents, you may need to go to court to become a conservator or guardian—a costly, public, and time-consuming process.

The Pro-Tip Solution: The "Big Three" Legal Documents. These must be created while your loved one still has "legal capacity"—the mental ability to understand the documents they are signing.

1. **Durable Power of Attorney (POA):**

• **What it is:** Designates an "agent" (you) to manage financial and legal affairs (paying bills, filing taxes, managing investments, selling property) when they become incapacitated.
• **Critical Detail:** Ensure it is "Durable," meaning it remains in effect after incapacity. A springing POA only "springs" into effect upon incapacity, which can require a doctor's certification and cause delays.

2. **Advanced Healthcare Directive (AHCD):** This is actually two documents in one.

• **Living Will:** Specifies wishes for end-of-life medical care (e.g., ventilator use, tube feeding).
• **Healthcare Power of Attorney (or Proxy):** Names a person to make all other medical decisions (e.g., choosing doctors, treatments, medications) when they cannot.

3. **Will and/or Living Trust:**

• **Will:** Dictates how assets are distributed after death.
• **Living Trust:** Holds assets during their lifetime and specifies how they are to be managed and distributed after death or incapacity. It avoids the public and often lengthy probate process.

Hidden Pitfall: The "Safe Deposit Box" Error. Once signed, these documents are useless if locked in a safe deposit box that no one else can access. Provide copies to your designated agents, your loved one's doctors, and your attorney. Keep the originals in a known, fireproof location at home.

Preparing Family Before Crisis: The "Family Meeting" Blueprint

The most common source of family conflict is not the disease itself, but the clash of expectations, old sibling rivalries, and the unequal distribution of caregiving labor. A proactive, structured family meeting is the antidote.

The Flawed Approach: Avoiding the conversation to "keep the peace." This guarantees a war later, when stress is high and decisions are urgent.

The Pro-Tip Solution: Facilitate a Formal Meeting.

•**Who:** All key family members, including the person with dementia if they are still in the early stages.
•**When:** As soon as possible after a diagnosis.
•**Goal:** To create a shared understanding and a unified plan.

Agenda for the First Meeting:

1.**Medical Update:** The primary caregiver or POA shares the diagnosis, prognosis, and what to expect.
2.**Financial Reality Check:** Present a clear picture of the loved one's assets, income, and insurance. Be transparent about the potential costs.
3.**Role Clarification:** Discuss and delegate roles based on skills and geography, not guilt.

•**The Local Primary:** Manages daily care, appointments.

•**The Financial Manager:** Handles bills, investments (often the POA agent).
•**The Researcher:** Looks into care options, benefits, legal aid.
•**The Communications Hub:** Keeps extended family and friends updated (e.g., via a private CaringBridge site).
4.**Define "Safe":** Discuss what "living at home" means and at what point it might become unsafe. Agree on the red flags that would trigger a move to a higher level of care.

Hidden Pitfall: The Long-Distance "Check-Writer." A sibling who contributes financially but is not involved in the day-to-day care may unintentionally undermine the primary caregiver's decisions. The primary caregiver's perspective on the urgency of a situation must be given the most weight.

When Living at Home is No Longer Safe: The Objective Red Flags

This is one of the most gut-wrenching decisions a family will make. Love and guilt scream, "Keep them home!" but safety must be the ultimate guide.

The Flawed Gauge: "We'll know when it's time." In the fog of daily care, the line is crossed gradually. What was unsafe yesterday becomes the "new normal" today.

The Pro-Tip Solution: Use an Objective Checklist. Don't rely on feelings; rely on facts.

Red Flags for Transition to a Higher Level of Care:

•**Wandering:** Any instance of leaving the home and getting lost, especially at night.
•**Fall Risk:** Multiple falls in a 6-month period, even if no major injury occurs.

- **Medication Mismanagement:** Inability to take medications correctly, leading to overdoses or missed doses with serious consequences.
- **Home Safety Hazards:** Leaving the stove on, causing small fires, flooding the bathroom.
- **Aggression or Paranoia:** Physical aggression toward the caregiver or extreme, constant suspicion that leads to unsafe situations.
- **Caregiver Collapse:** The health of the primary caregiver is deteriorating. **This is a valid and critical reason for a move.**
- **Incontinence:** Inability to manage toileting, leading to hygiene issues and high fall risk.
- **Social Isolation:** The person is no longer able to participate in any meaningful activity or social interaction at home; their world has shrunk to a single room.

Case Study: Robert's Choice - From Guilt to Grace

The Struggle: Robert, 70, promised his wife, Eleanor, he would never put her in a "home." For five years, he was her sole caregiver for Alzheimer's. He managed her incontinence, her agitation, and her sleepless nights. He was exhausted, isolated, and his own health was failing. His children saw the danger: Eleanor had started wandering, and Robert had fallen twice trying to help her at night. But when they suggested memory care, Robert erupted with guilt and grief. "I promised her!" he'd yell. The flawed solution of "toughing it out" was pushing the entire family toward a catastrophic breakdown.

The Turning Point: The crisis came when the police brought Eleanor home at 3 a.m.; she had wandered two miles in her nightgown. Sitting with his son the next day, Robert was shattered. His son didn't push. Instead, he reframed the problem. "Dad, you've kept your promise. You've cared for her at home longer and better than anyone could. But the disease has changed the rules. The promise now is to keep her safe. And right now, you're both in danger."

This reframe—from "breaking a promise" to "fulfilling a higher duty of safety"—was a lifeline for Robert. They visited a memory care facility together. Robert saw it wasn't a sterile "nursing home," but a secure, engaging community with trained staff. He saw residents listening to music and walking in secure gardens.

The Resolution: Robert moved Eleanor into memory care. The first month was filled with guilt, but he soon witnessed the change. Eleanor was safer, less agitated, and participating in music therapy. Robert, now freed from 24/7 vigilance, could finally rest. His visits transformed from a stressful chore to a joyful connection. He could be her husband again, holding her hand and talking about old times, instead of her exhausted nurse. He realized that by letting go of the literal interpretation of his promise, he had found a way to honor its spirit: to provide her with the best possible care and love, even if it looked different than he had originally imagined.

Conclusion

Confronting the financial, legal, and logistical realities of dementia is an act of profound love and courage. It requires difficult conversations and uncomfortable decisions made in the clear light of day, long before a crisis forces your hand. By creating a solid financial plan, establishing robust legal authority, fostering family unity, and defining objective safety benchmarks, you build a fortress of support around your loved one. This logistical groundwork does not replace compassion; it empowers it. It ensures that your energy can be focused on what matters most: providing love, comfort, and connection throughout the long and challenging journey ahead.

CHAPTER 8: Staying Connected Through Love & Memory: The Unbroken Bond

As Alzheimer's or another dementia progresses, it can feel as if the person you love is slipping away, piece by piece. The shared memories, the inside jokes, the very foundation of your relationship seems to be eroding. This chapter is not about reversing the disease, but about discovering something more profound: that the essence of a person, and the bond you share, can transcend the fragility of memory. We will explore powerful, evidence-based ways to connect with the feeling of the person, long after the facts of their life have faded. This is the territory where love becomes an action, not just a memory, and where we learn that the most powerful conversations often happen without words.

The Science of Connection: Bypassing the Intellect, Reaching the Heart

The Common Misconception: "If he doesn't remember me, our relationship is over. I've lost him."

The Interesting Angle/The Reality: While episodic memory (the "what, when, and where" of life) fades, the emotional memory often remains remarkably intact. The brain's limbic system, particularly the amygdala—the seat of emotion—is more resilient to the damage of Alzheimer's. This is why a person may not remember your name, but will still feel a sense of comfort, love, or joy in your presence. They are responding to the emotional truth of the moment, not the cognitive facts.

Pro-Tip: Shift Your Goal. The goal of a visit is no longer to elicit a specific memory ("Do you remember my wedding day?"). The new goal is to create a moment of shared positive emotion: a smile, a held hand, a sense of peace. You are not a historian; you are an emotional companion.

Hidden Pitfall: The Memory Test. Quizzing your loved one ("Who am I?" "What did you have for lunch?") only highlights their deficits, causing anxiety, shame, and withdrawal. It focuses on what is lost, guaranteeing a failed interaction for both of you.

Music Therapy & Familiar Melodies: The Soundtrack of the Self

Music is arguably the most powerful non-pharmacological tool for connection. Neurologist Oliver Sacks observed that music can "awake" people at every level of neurological impairment.

Why It Works: Music from a person's late teens and early twenties (between ages 15 and 25) is deeply hardwired into the brain's neural pathways. This "reminiscence bump" period is linked to identity formation, making these songs a direct line to a sense of self.

How to Use Music Effectively:

•**Create a "Life Soundtrack":** Compile a playlist of songs from their youth—the music they danced to, fell in love to, and worked to.

•**Set the Mood:** Use calming, familiar music (e.g., classical, big band) during meals or bath time to reduce anxiety. Use more upbeat music to encourage movement or joy.

•**Sing Together:** Don't worry about your voice. Singing familiar hymns, folk songs, or lullabies can elicit participation, even from those who rarely speak.

•**Focus on the Feeling:** Don't ask, "Do you remember this song?" Simply say, "I love this one," and listen together. Watch their face and body for a response—a tap of the finger, a hum, a relaxed posture.

> **A Moment of Connection:** Arthur, who had not spoken a coherent sentence in months, was sitting listlessly in his chair. His daughter put on Frank Sinatra's "I've Got You Under My Skin." As the horns swelled, Arthur's eyes closed. His fingers began to conduct an invisible orchestra. He didn't say a word, but for three minutes, he was no longer a man with dementia; he was a young man in a dance hall, full of life and rhythm. The music hadn't restored his memory; it had restored his essence.

The Power of Photos & Sensory Triggers: Speaking the Language of Sensation

As language fails, the senses become the primary mode of experiencing the world. We can use this to our advantage.

Photos Done Right:

•**Use Old Photos, Not Recent Ones:** A photo from their 30s or 40s is more likely to be recognized than one from last year.

•**Narrate, Don't Interrogate:** Instead of "Who is that?" try storytelling. "Look at this handsome couple. That's you and Mom on your wedding day. You look so happy." You are giving them a gift, not giving them a test.

•**Create a "Memory Box":** Fill a box with meaningful, tactile items: a favorite soft scarf, a well-worn baseball, a vintage perfume bottle, a stack of old letters. Let them hold and explore these objects. The feel and smell can trigger deep, non-verbal memories.

Engage the Senses:

•**Touch:** Give a hand massage with a familiar-scented lotion. Brush their hair. Offer a soft, textured blanket.
•**Smell:** Bake their favorite cookies. Bring in fresh-cut grass or the scent of pine. The olfactory nerve is directly connected to the memory and emotional centers of the brain.
•**Taste:** Share a simple, favorite food: a piece of chocolate, a strawberry, a bite of apple pie.

Simple Celebrations & Rituals: Finding Joy in the Present Moment

Large family holidays can be overwhelming and confusing. The noise, the crowd, and the broken expectations can lead to agitation and "sundowning."

Pro-Tip: Downscale and Adapt.

•**Celebrate in Micro-Moments:** Instead of a large Thanksgiving dinner, have a quiet lunch with just one or two people and a slice of pumpkin pie. The core element of the tradition—the taste—is preserved without the stress.
•**Focus on the Ritual, Not the Reason:** The comfort is in the familiar action, not the understanding of the event. Lighting a candle on a Friday night, having a pancake breakfast on Sunday, or watching a specific holiday movie can provide a deep sense of rhythm and security.
•**Celebrate the Person, Not the Date:** If a birthday party is too much, create a "You Are Loved" day. Bring flowers, play their music, and spend quiet, focused time with them. The celebration is of their continued presence in your life.

Religious & Cultural Traditions: The Comfort of the Familiar

For many, faith and cultural practices are a cornerstone of identity, offering a language of comfort that transcends cognitive understanding.

How to Incorporate Traditions:

- **Prayer & Hymns:** Reciting a familiar prayer (The Lord's Prayer, the Serenity Prayer) or singing a beloved hymn can be incredibly soothing. The words are stored in a different, more automatic part of the memory.
- **Ritual Objects:** The feel of rosary beads, the sight of a menorah, or the texture of a prayer rug can provide immense comfort.
- **Visits from Spiritual Leaders:** A familiar pastor, rabbi, or imam can be a welcome, calming presence, offering blessings and connection that feel deeply safe.
- **Cultural Foods & Language:** Speaking a few words in their native language or preparing a traditional dish can evoke a powerful sense of "home" and belonging.

> **A Moment of Connection:** Maria, whose mother had advanced dementia, was struggling to reach her. One day, in desperation, she began humming a lullaby in Spanish that her mother had sung to her as a child—"Duérmete, mi niña." Her mother, who had been nonverbal for weeks, stopped rocking. She turned her head, looked directly at Maria, and began to hum along. For a few minutes, they were connected not as patient and caregiver, but as mother and child, soothed by the ancient rhythm of love.

How Love Remains When Memory Fades: The Legacy of Feelings

This is the central, transformative truth of this chapter: **Love is not a memory; it is a felt experience.**

The person with dementia may forget your name, your face, and every specific thing you ever did together. But they are unlikely to forget the feeling you evoke. Are you a person who brings safety? Comfort? Joy? Patience? Or are you a person who brings stress, frustration, and pressure?

The love you have poured into them over a lifetime leaves a residue on their soul. It becomes part of their emotional landscape. When you sit with them in peaceful silence, when you hold their hand with tenderness, when you respond to their agitation with a calm voice, you are not just "managing behaviors." You are communicating love in its purest form—a form that does not require the messy translation of words or the perfect filing cabinet of memory.

Case Study: The Gift of Presence

The Struggle: David visited his father, Henry, every Sunday. For the first year after the diagnosis, these visits were agony. David would arrive with photos, trying to "jog" his father's memory. He'd talk about old times, growing increasingly frustrated and heartbroken when Henry stared back blankly. The visits felt like a failure, a weekly rehearsal of loss.

The Turning Point: A hospice social worker watched one of their interactions and gave David a simple piece of advice: "Stop trying to bring back the father you had. Just be with the father you have. Try just sitting with him. No talking. Just be."

The following Sunday, David was skeptical. He pulled a chair next to his father's, who was gazing out the window. He didn't bring out the photos. He didn't ask any questions. He simply sat, and after a while, he placed his hand over his father's. They sat in silence for twenty minutes, watching the trees sway in the wind. At one point, Henry, without turning his head, shifted his hand to grip David's.

The Resolution: That silent handhold was a more profound conversation than any they had had in years. David realized his father could no longer connect through stories, but he could still connect through presence. The love was still there, flowing in the silence. After that, David's visits changed. He would read the newspaper aloud, not caring if his father understood. He would play old jazz records. He would simply sit and be a loving presence. The pressure was gone. The grief remained, but it was now accompanied by a deep, abiding peace. David had learned the final, most difficult lesson of caregiving: how to love without requiring anything—not even recognition—in return. The journey through dementia is a process of continual letting go—of expectations, of shared narratives, of the person we once knew. But in that letting go, we can find a new way of being together. By speaking the language of the senses, of music, of touch, and of tranquil presence, we build a bridge to the soul that the disease cannot destroy. We learn that the ultimate connection is not based on the past we remember, but on the love we offer in the present moment. This love becomes our final, and most enduring, gift to them, and their final, unspoken gift to us.

CHAPTER 9: Self-Care for the Family: The Oxygen Mask Principle

The journey of caring for a loved one with dementia is often described as a "long goodbye." It is a marathon run on a track of quicksand, demanding every ounce of your physical, emotional, and spiritual energy. In this relentless process, the family caregiver is the most essential, and yet the most endangered, participant. This chapter confronts a truth that feels selfish but is in fact survivalist: you cannot pour from an empty cup. The well-being of the person you care for is inextricably linked to your own. We will navigate the treacherous terrain of caregiver stress and guilt, name the unique grief of mourning someone who is still here, and map a path for families to not only survive this journey, but to emerge with their bonds intact and their spirits resilient.

The Anatomy of Caregiver Burnout: More Than Just "Stress"

The Common Misconception: "I'm just tired. I'll sleep when this is over." or "Feeling this way means I'm not strong enough."

The Interesting Angle/The Reality: Caregiver burnout is not a personal failure or a sign of weak character. It is a **predictable and diagnosable state of physical, emotional, and mental exhaustion.** It is the direct result of an unsustainable situation, not a personal flaw.

Caption: Burnout is not a sudden event but a slow, insidious process. Recognizing your stage is the first step toward intervention.

Pro-Tip: The "Three-Sentence Check-In." Every day, ask yourself and answer honestly:

1. What is one thing I need **physically** right now? (e.g., a glass of water, a nap, a shower)
2. What is one thing I need **emotionally** right now? (e.g., a good cry, a laugh with a friend, five minutes of quiet)
3. What is one thing I need **spiritually** right now? (e.g., a walk in nature, a prayer, a moment of gratitude)

This practice forces you to tune into your own needs, breaking the cycle of self-neglect.

Hidden Pitfall: The "Superhero Complex." The belief that you are the only one who can provide proper care is a direct path to burnout. This mindset isolates you, pushes away potential help, and creates a single point of failure in the care system. The most competent caregivers are not superheroes; they are skilled managers who know how to delegate.

Managing the Tyranny of Guilt and Depression

Guilt is the caregiver's shadow, and depression is the storm that follows.

The Flawed Solution: "I just need to power through. My feelings don't matter right now."

Why It Fails: Suppressing emotions doesn't make them disappear; it forces them to manifest elsewhere—as explosive anger, somatic illness, or deep depression. Your feelings are not a distraction from the work; they are a critical part of it.

Strategies for Managing Guilt and Depression:
•**Reframe Guilt as a Signal:** Instead of letting guilt paralyze you, ask: "What is this guilt trying to tell me?" Guilt over taking time for yourself signals that you need to reaffirm that self-care is not selfish. Guilt over feeling angry signals that you need to find a healthy outlet for that frustration.
•**Practice "Both/And" Thinking:** The human heart is capable of holding conflicting emotions at once. You can be **both** deeply devoted to your loved one **and** utterly exhausted by the role. You can **both** love the person **and** hate the disease. Acknowledge the full spectrum of your experience.
•**Seek Professional Help:** Therapy is not a last resort; it is preventive maintenance for your mind. A therapist can provide tools for managing anxiety, reframing negative thought patterns, and processing the unique grief of caregiving. If you are experiencing persistent sadness, loss of interest in activities, changes in appetite or sleep, or thoughts of harming yourself, this is clinical depression, and you must seek help from a doctor or therapist.

The Emotional Journey of Grief Before Death: Ambiguous Loss

Dr. Pauline Boss's concept of **Ambiguous Loss** is the key to understanding the caregiver's grief. It is the most stressful form of loss because there is no closure.

•**Type 1:** The person is **physically absent but psychologically present** (e.g., a soldier missing in action).
•**Type 2 (The Caregiver's Experience):** The person is **physically present but psychologically absent.**

This creates a state of frozen grief. You are mourning the loss of the relationship, the shared future, and the person they were, all while they are still sitting in front of you. Society does not recognize your loss, so you are often left to grieve in isolation.

The Stages of this Unique Grief:

1. **Denial & Hope:** "Maybe it's just a phase. Maybe the new medication will bring them back."
2. **Hyper-Vigilance & Anxiety:** Trying to control the uncontrollable, constantly monitoring for safety.
3. **Anger & Resentment:** Anger at the disease, at other family members, at the world, and even at your loved one for leaving you in this impossible situation.
4. **Despair & Depression:** The full weight of the loss settles in. The person you knew is gone, and the work remains.
5. **Accommodation & Meaning-Making:** This is the goal. It is not "acceptance" in a happy sense, but a reorganization of your life and identity to find a new way forward. You learn to love the person who is here, while holding space for the person who is gone.

Pro-Tip: Rituals of Release. Create small, private rituals to acknowledge your grief. Write a letter to the person your loved one used to be and burn it safely. Light a candle in their honor. Visit a place that was special to you both and speak your grief aloud. This gives your loss a tangible outlet.

How Families Can Heal and Stay United

Dementia can tear families apart, or it can become the crucible that forges them stronger. The difference lies in intentional strategy.

The Most Common Flawed Solution: The "Designated Martyr" dynamic, where one person does everything, siblings criticize from afar, and communication breaks down into a blame game.

The Pro-Tip Solution: The Family Care Contract.

Hold a formal family meeting, facilitated by a neutral third party (a therapist, clergy member, or geriatric care manager) if necessary. The goal is to move from assumption to agreement.

The Contract Should Cover:

1.**Role Definition:** Who is the primary point of contact for doctors? Who manages finances? Who is the "researcher"? Who provides respite? Assign roles based on skills and geography, not guilt.
2.**Communication Protocol:** How will updates be shared? (e.g., a private family group chat or a CaringBridge site). How often will you check in as a group?
3.**Financial Transparency:** The primary caregiver must be open about costs, and the family must agree on a budget and how to handle expenses. The long-distance sibling who cannot provide hands-on care can often contribute financially.
4.**Conflict Resolution:** Agree in advance: "When we disagree, we will focus on the problem, not attack the person. We will remember that we are all on the same team, and the enemy is the disease, not each other."

Case Study: The Sanchez Family - From Fractured to Fortified

The Struggle: After their father's Alzheimer's diagnosis, the three Sanchez siblings fell into classic roles. Maria, the oldest and local, became the sole caregiver. Carlos, the middle child, sent money but criticized Maria's decisions from across the country. Elena, the youngest, was "too busy" with her young family to be involved. Maria grew resentful, Carlos felt guilty and defensive, and Elena was completely shut out. Family calls were tense and unproductive.

The Turning Point: The crisis came when Maria was hospitalized with severe exhaustion. With no plan in place, Carlos had to fly in urgently, and Elena was forced to step in. The chaos was a wake-up call. At Maria's kitchen table, still pale from her hospital stay, she said, "We can't do this anymore. We are failing Dad and we are destroying our family."

They decided to create a "Family Care Contract." They defined roles: Maria remained the day-to-day manager, but Carlos took over all financial and insurance paperwork. Elena, though distant, became the official "Communications Director," providing weekly updates to the extended family and coordinating a schedule for respite care contributions from cousins. They agreed to a monthly video call to discuss decisions, with a rule: "No blaming, only problem-solving."

The Resolution: The contract did not erase the stress, but it gave them a structure to manage it. Maria felt seen and supported for the first time. Carlos felt connected and useful beyond just writing a check. Elena re-engaged, finding small but meaningful ways to contribute. They began to share funny stories about their dad in their group chat, rediscovering the bond that had been buried under the weight of the disease. They learned that unity wasn't about agreeing on everything, but about committing to the shared mission of caring for their father and each other.

Conclusion

The path of the family caregiver is one of the most challenging any human can walk. It will test your limits, your patience, and your heart. But within this struggle lies a profound opportunity for growth. By treating your own well-being as non-negotiable, by honoring the complex grief you carry, and by intentionally forging a united family front, you do more than just survive. You learn the deepest lessons of compassion, resilience, and love. You discover that the oxygen mask principle is not a metaphor for selfishness, but for survival. By securing your own mask first, you ensure you have the strength, clarity, and heart to help the person you love until the very end of the journey. And in doing so, you heal not only them, but yourself.

CHAPTER 10: Real-Life Case Studies: Lessons from the Front Lines

Dementia is not a single story. It is a collection of millions of individual narratives, each with its own unique characters, conflicts, and moments of grace. While medical textbooks describe the pathology of the disease, it is within the lived experiences of families that we find the true meaning of care, love, and resilience. This chapter presents five unvarnished stories from the front lines of dementia care. These are not tales of perfect families, but of real people navigating imperfect situations. Within their struggles and their solutions lie the most practical and profound lessons for anyone on this path.

Case Study 1: The Husband – "In Sickness and In Health"

The Characters: Arthur, 78, a retired engineer; Eleanor, 76, his wife of 55 years, diagnosed with Alzheimer's.

The Story: Arthur was a problem-solver. He approached Eleanor's diagnosis like one of his engineering projects: with spreadsheets, schedules, and unwavering determination. For the first three years, he managed everything—the medications, the meals, the finances—priding himself on his efficiency. He refused his children's offers of help, believing it was his sacred duty, his promise, to care for her alone.

The Crisis: The crisis was not a single event but a slow, insidious erosion. Arthur's own health began to fail under the 24/7 strain. He developed hypertension and crippling back pain from assisting Eleanor. The man who was once patient began to snap at her when she repeated questions for the tenth time, followed by waves of crushing guilt. The turning point came when he forgot to give Eleanor her heart medication for three days, a mistake his "perfect" system was designed to prevent.

The Solution: Arthur's daughter, Sarah, intervened not with criticism, but with a partnership. She didn't say, "You're doing it wrong." She said, "Let me be your assistant. Train me on your system." She spent a weekend learning his methods, then gently introduced tools to reduce his cognitive load: a automated pill dispenser, a pre-paid grocery delivery service, and a commitment from a home health aide for four hours, twice a week, to give him a guaranteed break.

The Lesson: Arthur learned that his marriage vow, "in sickness and in health," did not mean "in isolation and to the point of self-destruction." By accepting help, he was not breaking his promise; he was ensuring he could keep it with love and patience, rather than exhaustion and resentment. He transitioned from being a solitary caregiver to the CEO of Eleanor's care team, preserving his own health so he could be her husband for longer.

Case Study 2: The Two Sisters – "The Proximity Guilt Divide"

The Characters: Linda, 62, a local schoolteacher; Karen, 58, a corporate lawyer living a three-hour flight away; their mother, Rose, with vascular dementia.

The Story: Linda, living closest to their mother, naturally fell into the primary caregiver role. Karen sent money and called weekly, offering advice from a distance. Resentment festered. Linda felt Karen's financial contributions were a "cop-out," buying her way out of the hard, daily work. Karen felt Linda was controlling and dismissed her ideas without consideration.

Their phone calls became battlegrounds, rehashing childhood rivalries.

The Crisis: A fall sent Rose to the hospital. Linda, overwhelmed, called Karen in a panic. Karen flew in and immediately began questioning every decision Linda had made —the doctor's choice, the medication, the state of the house. A massive argument erupted in the hospital hallway, leaving both sisters in tears and their mother's discharge plan in limbo.

The Solution: A hospital social worker mediated a conversation. She had each sister answer one question: "What is your biggest fear for your mother?" Both answered, "That she won't get the best care." The social worker then reframed their conflict: "You both want the same thing. You are just speaking different languages: the language of daily hands-on care and the language of long-distance advocacy." They created a written "Partnership Pact." Linda was the "Care Commander," with final say on daily decisions. Karen was the "Finance and Research Officer," responsible for managing bills and investigating long-term care options. They agreed to a weekly, structured video call with a set agenda.

The Lesson: Geographic proximity often dictates caregiving roles, but it does not dictate caregiving love. Conflict often stems from unspoken expectations and different "languages" of care. Formalizing roles and establishing structured communication can transform adversarial relationships into complementary partnerships.

Case Study 3: The Long-Distance Child – "The Remote Project Manager"

The Characters: Mark, 45, a tech executive in Singapore; his father, David, 80, living alone in London after a recent dementia diagnosis.

The Story: Mark was plagued by worry and guilt from 7,000 miles away. Phone calls with his father were increasingly confusing. Bills were going unpaid, and the fridge was often empty. David insisted he was fine, refusing to acknowledge any problems. Mark felt helpless and terrified, trying to manage a crisis from another continent.

The Crisis: David was found wandering his neighborhood in his pajedes at 2 a.m. by a neighbor who called Mark. It was clear that living alone was no longer safe, and Mark had to act immediately.

The Solution: Mark became a "remote care CEO." He hired a local geriatric care manager (GCM) in London to be his "eyes and ears." The GCM conducted a full assessment, facilitated difficult conversations with David, and vetted memory care facilities. Mark used technology to stay connected: he set up a digital picture frame that he could send photos to remotely, scheduled weekly video calls facilitated by an aide, and used a shared calendar app with the GCM to track appointments and medication changes.

The Lesson: Physical distance does not equal emotional absence. Effective long-distance caregiving is not about doing everything yourself, but about strategically deploying and managing local resources. A geriatric care manager is an invaluable investment for a long-distance caregiver, providing professional, on-the-ground oversight and peace of mind.

Case Study 4: The Grandchildren – "Why Is Grandma Scary?"

The Characters: Liam, 8, and his sister Chloe, 11; their grandmother, "Nana" Patricia, who had frontotemporal dementia, which caused uncharacteristic outbursts and loss of social filters.

The Story: Liam and Chloe were very close to their fun, cookie-baking Nana. As her disease progressed, she began saying cruel, inappropriate things, would get angry over minor changes, and sometimes didn't seem to recognize them. Chloe became withdrawn, making excuses not to visit. Liam started having nightmares and became clingy with his parents.

The Crisis: During a family birthday party, Patricia loudly accused Chloe of stealing her purse. When the purse was found in another room, she showed no remorse. Chloe ran to her room, sobbing, "I hate her! She's a monster!"

The Solution: The children's parents sat them down for a "family meeting." They used the "sick brain" analogy, explaining, "Nana's brain has a sickness that sometimes makes the words come out wrong. It makes her feel scared and angry inside, and that comes out at us. It's like a computer glitch. It's not her, and it's definitely not because of anything you did." They gave the children new, safe "jobs." Liam's job was to be the "Official Greeter" (a simple wave and hello). Chloe's job was to be the "Head of Music," choosing songs to play for Nana. They also instituted a "safe word"—"banana"—that either child could say to signal they needed an immediate break from the visit, no questions asked.

The Lesson: Children need a developmentally appropriate explanation for behavioral changes. Without it, they will internalize the blame or become fearful. By giving them a medical framework and empowering them with controlled, low-pressure ways to interact, you can protect their emotional well-being and preserve a modified, but meaningful, connection.

Case Study 5: Late-Stage Care – "The Peaceful Letting Go"

The Characters: The entire Miller family; their matriarch, Helen, 89, in the final stages of Alzheimer's, non-verbal and bedridden in home hospice care.

The Story: For a decade, the family had fought the disease, focusing on safety, stimulation, and medication. Now, the goal was shifting from active care to comfort care. This was a difficult mental transition for some family members, who felt that "giving up" on curative measures was a betrayal.

The Crisis: Helen developed pneumonia, a common end-of-life complication. Some family members insisted she be rushed to the hospital for antibiotics. Others, guided by hospice, felt she should be kept comfortable at home. The family was divided at the most vulnerable moment.

The Solution: The hospice nurse gathered the family. She gently explained that transferring a late-stage dementia patient to the hospital is often more traumatic than comforting, involving needles, unfamiliar faces, and invasive procedures. She reframed their goal: "Our job now is not to prolong her dying, but to ensure her peace." They created a vigil schedule so Helen was never alone. They played her favorite classical music, massaged her hands with lavender lotion, and spoke to her, sharing loving memories and giving her permission to let go. The focus was entirely on comfort, presence, and love.

The Lesson: The final stage of care is not about surrender; it is about a profound shift in intention. It is the transition from "doing everything" to "being everything"—being a peaceful, loving presence. Hospice care provides the medical and emotional support to facilitate a dignified and gentle passing, honoring a life well-lived rather than fighting a battle that can no longer be won. In the end, the family found that their shared vigil, though heartbreaking, was also deeply unifying and healing.

These five stories illustrate that there is no one "right" way to navigate dementia. The path is different for a husband, for sisters, for a long-distance son, for grandchildren, and for a family at the end of life. Yet, common threads run through them all: the danger of isolation, the necessity of clear communication, the power of redefining roles, and the ultimate truth that love must often express itself through practicality, patience, and the courage to accept help. By learning from these real-life journeys, we can face our own with greater wisdom, compassion, and resilience.

Here is a detailed breakdown of the most common flawed solutions and why they are ultimately ineffective.

The Flawed Logic of Common Dementia "Fixes"

The core reason these solutions fail is that they are designed for a **cognitively intact brain**. They rely on logic, memory, and self-control—precisely the faculties that dementia dismantles. Applying these solutions is like trying to use a manual for a car to fix a boat; the fundamental operating system is different.

1. The Solution: "Correcting Them and Re-Orienting Them to Reality"

•**What it looks like:** "Mom, I told you already, your mother passed away 20 years ago." "No, Dad, today is Tuesday, not Saturday." "You don't live there anymore, remember we moved you here?"
•**The Flawed Logic:** "If I just give them the correct information, they will remember and understand. It's my job to keep them grounded in reality."
•**Why It Doesn't Work & Makes Things Worse:**

•**It Attacks Their Reality:** The person with dementia lives in a subjective, often confusing reality. Correcting them directly challenges their perception of the world, which is one of the few things they have left. This doesn't bring them into your reality; it isolates them in theirs, making them feel attacked, stupid, and defensive.
•**It Causes "Catastrophic Reactions":** This constant correction is a primary trigger for anxiety, agitation, and anger. Being told you are wrong about fundamental facts is profoundly threatening.
•**It Erodes Trust and Self-Esteem:** The person learns that interacting with you is a source of humiliation and failure, so they may withdraw entirely.

The Effective Alternative: Validation Therapy. Enter their reality. If they are waiting for their mother, don't state the fact of her death. Instead, connect with the emotion: "You must miss your mother a lot. Tell me about her." You are validating the feeling (longing, love), not the faulty fact.

2. The Solution: "Using Logic and Reason to Stop Repetitive Questions"

•**What it looks like:** "Dad, we have discussed this five times. The doctor's appointment is at 2 p.m. tomorrow. I've written it down. Please stop asking."
•**The Flawed Logic:** "If I provide a clear, logical answer and even evidence (a note), they will retain the information and the behavior will stop."
•**Why It Doesn't Work & Makes Things Worse:**

•**The Memory Gate is Broken:** The issue isn't a lack of information; it's that the brain cannot hold onto new information. The question is forgotten almost as soon as it's asked, but the underlying anxiety remains. The repetition is a symptom of that anxiety, not a cognitive choice.
•**It Fuels Caregiver Resentment:** The caregiver expends immense energy repeating the same logical answer, only to be asked again moments later. This leads to frustration, sarcasm, and yelling, which only frightens the person.
•**It Misses the Real Need:** The repetitive question "What are we doing today?" is rarely about the schedule. It's a cry for reassurance, a way to combat the terrifying feeling of uncertainty and lost control.

The Effective Alternative: Address the Emotion, Not the Question. Provide reassurance instead of information. "Everything is taken care of. You're safe here with me. How about we have a cup of tea?" Often, satisfying the underlying need for security stops the cycle.

3. The Solution: "Expecting Them to Remember and Follow Instructions"

•**What it looks like:** "I told you to get dressed after breakfast. Why are you still in your pajamas?" "Please go into the living room and bring me my reading glasses."
•**The Flawed Logic:** "They should be able to follow a simple, one- or two-step command. They are just being stubborn or lazy."
•**Why It Doesn't Work & Makes Things Worse:**

•**Executive Function is Impaired:** Dementia damages the brain's "CEO"—the part that plans, sequences, and initiates tasks. "Get dressed" is not one task; it's a complex sequence: choose clothes, take off pajamas, put on underwear, pants, shirt, etc. The brain gets lost in the steps.
•**It Sets Them Up for Failure:** You are asking them to perform a task their brain is physically incapable of completing. This leads to frustration and a sense of incompetence.
•**It Creates Unnecessary Conflict:** The caregiver interprets the inaction as defiance, leading to arguments over a biological impossibility.

The Effective Alternative: "Show, Don't Tell." Break tasks down into single, concrete steps and initiate them together. Instead of "Get dressed," try: "Here is your shirt. Let's put your arm in this sleeve." Or better yet, use visual cues by starting the task alongside them.

4. The Solution: "Asking Open-Ended Questions or Testing Their Memory"

•**What it looks like:** "What did you do this morning?" "Do you remember what we had for lunch?" "Who is that in this photograph?"

•**The Flawed Logic:** "I need to keep their mind active and engaged. Asking questions will stimulate their memory."
•**Why It Doesn't Work & Makes Things Worse:**

•**It's a Pop Quiz They Always Fail:** These questions require the person to access recent or remote memory, which is compromised. Every failed question is a small reminder of their cognitive losses, chipping away at their personhood.
•**It Creates Pressure and Anxiety:** The person feels put on the spot, which can shut down communication entirely.
•**It Hinders, Not Helps, Connection:** The interaction becomes a test rather than a conversation.

The Effective Alternative: Use Statements and Shared Observations. Instead of "What did you do?", say "I heard you listened to some lovely music this morning." Instead of "Who is this?", narrate the photo: "This is a picture of you and your brother at the lake. You both loved to fish." You are sharing the memory, not demanding it.

5. The Solution: "The Primary Caregiver Handling Everything Themselves to Protect the Loved One"

•**What it looks like:** A spouse or adult child refuses all offers of help, insisting, "I'm the only one who knows how to care for them," or "A stranger would just confuse and upset them."
•**The Flawed Logic:** "My love and dedication are the best care. Involving others will cause more stress than it's worth. It's my duty to do this alone."
•**Why It Doesn't Work & Makes Things Worse:**

•**It's a Single-Point-of-Failure System:** This is the most predictable path to caregiver burnout. When the sole caregiver becomes exhausted, depressed, or physically ill, the entire care structure collapses, leading to a crisis that is far more traumatic for the person with dementia.

•It Robs the Loved One of Potential Comfort: While change is hard, a new, calm caregiver can often connect in different, positive ways without the emotional baggage of a long history.
•It Creates Resentment: The caregiver, though acting from love, will inevitably grow to resent the immense, unshared burden. This resentment poisons the very relationship they are trying to protect.

The Effective Alternative: The "Care Manager" Model. The most loving and strategic thing a primary caregiver can do is to transition from being the sole "doer" to the "manager" of a care team. This involves gradually introducing help in small, positive doses and building a sustainable system that ensures consistent, loving care even when the primary caregiver needs a break.

The Paradigm Shift

The common thread is that these flawed solutions are **caregiver-centric**. They are about trying to force the person with dementia to fit into our world of logic, time, and memory. The solutions that actually work require a **person-centered** paradigm shift: we must be the ones to adapt. We must learn to speak the language of emotion, to live in their moment, and to connect with the person who remains, rather than fighting the disease by trying to restore the person who is gone. This shift is the difference between a daily battle and a journey of compassionate connection.

are they solving the problems ? if so , how?

> This is the most important question. The "flawed solutions" **do not solve the core problem—the progression of the dementia itself.** However, to be fair, they are often deployed to solve a different, more immediate set of problems for the **caregiver**.

Let's break down what these common fixes are attempting to solve and how they provide a temporary, illusionary sense of success before ultimately failing.

What the Flawed Solutions Are Trying to Solve:

1. **For the Caregiver's Anxiety and Helplessness:** When a loved one lives in a different reality, it is deeply unsettling. Correcting them ("That person is dead," "Today is Tuesday") is an attempt by the caregiver to **anchor themselves**. It's a way of shouting into the void, "My world is still real and logical!" It provides a fleeting moment of control in a situation that is fundamentally out of control.
2. **For the Caregiver's Exhaustion and Frustration:** Answering the same question for the tenth time is maddening. Using logic and reason is an attempt to **achieve efficiency**. The caregiver is desperately trying to close a frustrating loop. They think, "If I can just make the information stick this time, I can get some mental relief."
3. **For the Caregiver's Grief and Fear:** Asking memory-testing questions ("Do you remember who I am?") is often a desperate, heart-wrenching attempt to **grab hold of the person who is slipping away**. For one fleeting second, if the loved one answers correctly, the caregiver gets a hit of the "old" person. It's not about stimulating the patient's brain; it's about soothing the caregiver's breaking heart.
4. **For the Caregiver's Sense of Duty and Love:** The "I'll do it all myself" martyrdom is an attempt to **fulfill a profound emotional promise** ("in sickness and in health"). It feels like the ultimate expression of love and dedication. Saying "I can

handle it" is a way to maintain a pre-disease identity as a capable, loving spouse or child.

How They "Work" in the Short Term (The Illusion of Success):

- **They Provide a Sense of Control:** Correcting someone or giving a logical answer makes the caregiver feel, for a moment, like they are "managing" the situation. It's an active response to a passive, terrifying decline.
- **They Release Pent-Up Frustration:** Snapping, "I already told you that!" provides a cathartic release for the caregiver's built-up stress, even though it's immediately followed by guilt.
- **They Offer a Moment of Connection (False Positive):** On the rare occasion a memory test works ("Yes, you're my daughter!"), it provides a powerful, euphoric moment of reconnection that reinforces the flawed behavior.
- **They Uphold a Self-Image:** Playing the heroic, self-sacrificing caregiver can be a source of identity and pride, until it leads to collapse.

Why They Ultimately Fail as Real Solutions:

Because they solve the caregiver's temporary emotional needs at the direct expense of the person with dementia's core, long-term needs.

A real solution is one that improves the well-being and quality of life for **both** parties over the long haul. The flawed solutions do the opposite:

Flawed Solution	What It Solves for Caregiver (Short-Term)	What It Does to the Person with Dementia (Long-Term)	The Net Result
Correcting & Re-Orienting	Provides a sense of control, upholds "reality."	Causes anxiety, shame, and erosion of trust.	**Increased distress for both; broken relationship.**
Using Logic & Reason	Provides catharsis, feels efficient.	Confuses, agitates, and fails to address underlying fear.	**Caregiver is more frustrated; loved one is more anxious.**
Memory Testing	Offers a fleeting moment of hope and connection.	Highlights disability, causes humiliation and withdrawal.	**Caregiver's heartbreak is prolonged; loved one retreats.**
Martyrdom ("I'll do it all")	Fulfills a sense of duty and identity.	Creates a fragile care system and isolates the loved one.	**Total system collapse (caregiver burnout), leading to**

Flawed Solution	What It Solves for Caregiver (Short-Term)	What It Does to the Person with Dementia (Long-Term)	The Net Result
			crisis.

How the Effective Alternatives Actually Solve the Problem:

The successful strategies shift the goal from **controlling the disease** to **managing the relationship and environment**. They work because they are aligned with the **actual, current capabilities** of the brain with dementia.

1. **Validation Therapy solves the problem of disconnection.** By joining their reality, you are not "giving in to the disease"; you are **building a bridge of trust**. This reduces the loved one's anxiety and makes them more cooperative and less agitated, which in turn reduces the caregiver's stress. It solves the problem of conflict.
2. **Addressing the emotion behind repetitive questions solves the problem of exhaustion.** By providing reassurance instead of information, you **extinguish the anxiety fueling the loop**. The questions stop because the underlying need is met. This saves the caregiver's sanity and calms the loved one. It solves the problem of endless, frustrating repetition.

3. **"Show, Don't Tell" solves the problem of task failure.** By breaking down tasks and initiating them, you are **providing cognitive scaffolding**. You are using the parts of their brain that still work (procedural memory, the ability to mimic) to bypass the parts that don't (executive function). This gets the task done without a fight. It solves the problem of daily care battles.
4. **Building a care team solves the problem of systemic collapse.** It recognizes that dementia is a marathon. By delegating, the primary caregiver **preserves their own health and capacity to love**, which is the single most valuable resource the loved one has. It solves the problem of long-term sustainability.

In summary:

The flawed solutions are **palliative for the caregiver's emotions** but **toxic to the care recipient's well-being**. They are like drinking saltwater to quench a thirst—it seems to help for a second but ultimately makes the situation much, much worse.

The effective solutions are **therapeutic for the relationship**. They acknowledge that the only thing you can truly control is your own approach. By changing your behavior to fit their needs, you create a calmer, safer, and more loving environment for everyone involved. That is how you actually solve the solvable problems of dementia care.

PART 2

-Is alzheimers disease hereditary ?

-How to Care for Someone with Alzheimers Disease ?

-What are the Symptoms of Alzheimers Disease ?

-How Doctors Diagnose Alzheimers Disease ?

-How to Prevent Early Alzheimer ?

-How to Prevent Alzheimer Disease Naturally?

-What's the Difference Between Alzheimer's & Dementia ?

-What causes dementia ?

-Medical Care for Alzheimers

Is Alzheimer's Disease Hereditary?

1-Is Alzheimer's Disease Hereditary? The Gene Story, Simplified

The short answer is: Yes, genetics can play a role, but the story has two very different parts. For most people, the disease is not a simple, pre-determined genetic fate.

The fear that Alzheimer's is a straight line of inheritance from parent to child is one of the biggest sources of anxiety. The empowering truth is that for the vast majority of cases, genes only influence your risk; they don't dictate your destiny.

To understand this, we need to talk about two types of genetic influence: Familial Alzheimer's Disease (FAD) and Late-Onset Alzheimer's Disease.

1. Familial Alzheimer's Disease (FAD): The Rare, Hereditary Form

•**What it is:** This is a very rare, inherited form of Alzheimer's, caused by a single specific genetic mutation. It accounts for **less than 1%** of all Alzheimer's cases.
•**The Genetics:** If a parent has a mutation in one of three specific genes (the APP, PSEN1, or PSEN2 genes), each of their children has a **50/50 chance** of inheriting it.
•**The Hallmark: Early Onset.** This form almost always develops before age 65, often in a person's 40s or 50s. The progression is often more rapid.
•**The Bottom Line:** If FAD runs in your family, the disease is strongly hereditary. This is often confirmed when multiple

generations and several family members are diagnosed at a young age.

2. Late-Onset Alzheimer's: The Common, "Risk-Influenced" Form

This is the most common form of the disease, accounting for over **95%** of all cases, typically occurring after age 65.

•**The Key Player: The APOE Gene.** Here, the story shifts from deterministic genes to risk genes. The most significant known genetic risk factor is a gene called **Apolipoprotein E (APOE)**.

•Everyone has two copies of the APOE gene (one from each parent).
•It comes in three common forms (alleles): ε2, ε3, and ε4.
•**APOE-ε3** is the most common and is considered neutral.
•**APOE-ε2** is relatively rare and is thought to be somewhat protective.
•**APOE-ε4** is the risk factor. Having one copy of ε4 (from one parent) increases your risk. Having two copies (from both parents) increases your risk even more.

It is critical to understand what this means:

•**Having the APOE-ε4 gene does NOT mean you will get Alzheimer's.** Many people with the ε4 allele never develop the disease.
•**Not having the APOE-ε4 gene does NOT mean you are immune.** Many people diagnosed with Alzheimer's have no ε4 alleles.

•**A Large Slice (Estimated 60-70%): Lifestyle & Environmental Factors.** This includes diet, exercise, sleep,

cardiovascular health, education, and social engagement. **This is the part you can influence.**
•**A Smaller Slice (30-40%): Genetics.** This includes the APOE gene and other yet-to-be-discovered risk genes.
•**A Tiny Slice (<1%): Strongly Hereditary (FAD) Mutations.**

The Empowering Reframe: Genetics Loads the Gun, Lifestyle Pulls the Trigger

This common saying in medicine is perfectly applicable to Alzheimer's. Your genes (like APOE-ε4) may predispose you, but your lifestyle choices are what largely determine whether that predisposition becomes a reality.

What This Means For You:

1. **If You Have a Family History of Late-Onset Alzheimer's:** You may have an increased genetic risk, but you are not powerless. This knowledge should be a motivator to double down on the modifiable risk factors within your control.
2. **If You Have a Family History of Early-Onset (FAD):** This is a much more serious genetic link. Genetic counseling is highly recommended for families with this history to understand the risks and options.

Pro-Tips and Hidden Pitfalls

•**Pro-Tip: Focus on Your "Controllables."** Regardless of your family history, the most powerful actions you can take are the same:

•**Prioritize Heart Health:** What's good for your heart is good for your brain. Manage blood pressure, cholesterol, and blood sugar.
•**Get Moving:** Regular aerobic exercise is one of the most potent, evidence-based strategies for brain health.
•**Nourish Your Brain:** Follow a MIND or Mediterranean diet, rich in plants, berries, and healthy fats.
•**Stay Connected:** Social engagement and continuous learning build "cognitive reserve."
•**Hidden Pitfall: Genetic Determinism.** The belief that "it's all in my genes" can lead to fatalism and inaction. The research is clear: a healthy lifestyle can significantly reduce your risk, even if you carry the APOE-ε4 gene. One study showed that people with a high genetic risk who followed a favorable lifestyle had a **55% lower risk** of developing dementia than those with an unfavorable lifestyle.
•**Hidden Pitfall: Direct-to-Consumer Genetic Testing Anxiety.** Companies like 23andMe can tell you your APOE status. It is crucial to speak with a doctor or genetic counselor before taking such a test to understand what the results can and cannot tell you. A positive result for ε4 can cause significant anxiety without changing the recommended, healthy lifestyle actions.

A Story of Empowerment, Not Fear

Maria watched her grandmother and then her father struggle with Alzheimer's. She spent years living in fear, convinced a ticking time bomb was inside her. "It's inevitable," she'd say, avoiding articles and conversations about the disease.

When her own memory lapses began in her 50s, her fear turned to paralysis. Finally, her doctor asked her a transformative question: "Maria, instead of waiting for the disease, what if you started building your defenses today?"

This reframe changed everything. Maria didn't get genetic testing; she started building her "cognitive reserve." She joined a walking group (exercise and social connection). She took a cooking class to learn the Mediterranean diet (nutrition and cognitive challenge). She began managing her stress with yoga.

She hasn't just been waiting; she's been building. The shadow of heredity is still there, but it's now countered by the tangible strength of her daily habits. She understands that her family history isn't a life sentence; it's a warning sign that has empowered her to take the wheel. She is actively writing a different ending for her own story.

While a rare form of Alzheimer's is directly hereditary, the common form is not. Your risk is influenced by a complex interplay of genetics and lifestyle. This is ultimately empowering news: the daily choices you make about how you live, eat, move, and think are your most powerful weapons in protecting your brain's future.

How to Care for Someone With Alzheimer's Disease

Caring for someone with Alzheimer's is one of the most challenging responsibilities a family can face. It is a journey that changes day by day, sometimes hour by hour. Alzheimer's is unpredictable—some days are calm and clear, and others are filled with confusion, agitation, or fear. Effective care is not just about feeding and bathing. It is about **communication, safety, dignity, emotional support, and patience.**

This section will show caregivers **how to take care of the mind, body, and emotions** of someone living with Alzheimer's — while protecting their own health too.

✅A Real Story

Thomas, a 78-year-old grandfather, used to read the newspaper every morning. One day, he woke up angry, accusing his wife of hiding it. She tried to explain he already read it, but he became frustrated and yelled. She argued with him, insisted he was wrong, and tried to make him remember.

The more she explained, the worse he got.
He threw the remote, cried, and locked himself in the bedroom.

Later, a dementia specialist told her something life-changing:

**"You don't win with logic in Alzheimer's.
You win with calm, redirection, and emotion."**

When Thomas became confused again, instead of arguing, she sat beside him and said,
"I'm sorry that upset you. Let's read together."
He relaxed. The anger disappeared.

? **Lesson:** Alzheimer's patients respond to emotion, not logic.

✅Understanding the Alzheimer's Care Model

There are three pillars of care:

```
1. Safety        → Prevent dangers, create
calm spaces
2. Routine       → Daily structure reduces
confusion
3. Communication → Speak in simple,
reassuring ways
```

If you get these three right, the home becomes peaceful instead of stressful.

✅1. Creating a Safe Home Environment

Alzheimer's reduces judgment, coordination, memory, and awareness of danger.

A home that seems normal to you can be dangerous to them.

✅Home Safety Checklist (Practical)

Area	What Can Go Wrong	What To Do
Kitchen	Burning food, leaving gas on, eating spoiled items	Remove gas knobs, lock chemicals, keep microwave meals only
Bathroom	Slipping, drowning risk, confusion with faucets	Non-slip mats, grab bars, simple faucets
Bedroom	Wandering at night, falls	Motion-sensor lights, bed rails, clear pathways
Doors	Leaving the house, getting lost	Install door alarms or childproof locks
General	Clutter, loose rugs, stairs	Remove tripping hazards, install handrails

✅Fast safety fixes that help instantly:

- Replace sharp knives with safer options
- Label drawers with pictures (not words)
- Use big clocks & large calendars
- Keep dangerous medicines locked

✅2. The Power of Routine

People with Alzheimer's lose memory, but their brain responds well to **pattern**.

A predictable schedule reduces anxiety because:

- They know what happens next
- Their brain doesn't struggle with decisions
- Behavior problems decrease

✅ **Sample Daily Routine Chart**

Time	Activity
7:00	Wake up, bathroom, morning medication
7:30	Breakfast (same seat every day)
9:00	Light exercise / walk
10:00	Simple activities (puzzles, folding towels)
12:30	Lunch
1:30	Nap or quiet time
3:00	Music, TV, or family time
6:00	Dinner
8:30	Bath, bedtime routine

Why this works: Familiar patterns reduce confusion, prevent agitation, and help sleep.

✅ **3. Communication that Works**

Talking to someone with Alzheimer's requires special strategy.

✅ **What DOESN'T Work**

❌Arguing
❌Asking "Do you remember?"
❌Giving long explanations
❌Correcting their mistakes
❌Speaking fast or loud

✅ **What DOES Work**

✅ Short sentences
✅ Calm, friendly tone
✅ Eye contact & gentle touch
✅ One instruction at a time
✅ Offering choices ("Tea or juice?" not "What do you want?")

Here is an effective method professionals use:

✅The "3-second Rule"

Say something, then wait **3 seconds**.
Their brain needs more time to process.

✅How to Deal With Difficult Behaviors

Alzheimer's can cause:

- Wandering
- Repeating questions
- Accusing family of stealing
- Night confusion
- Anger or crying
- Refusing to bathe or eat

✅The Behavior Reaction Formula

```
BEHAVIOR = Communication of a need
```

They are not difficult — they are **trying to communicate**.

✅Chart: Behavior Causes

Behavior	Possible Cause	What Helps
Yelling / anger	Fear, confusion, overstimulation	Speak softly, move to quiet space
Wandering	Boredom, need to pee, hunger	Short walks, bathroom schedule
Repeating questions	Anxiety, insecurity	Answer calmly, distraction
Refusing bath	Embarrassment, cold water	Warm bathroom, calm music, privacy

Behavior	Possible Cause	What Helps
Accusing stealing	Memory loss of where items were placed	Duplicates of common items, secure storage

✅ **Example: Repeating Questions**

Instead of:
❌ "I told you already!"
❌ "How many times must I answer?"

Try:
✅ "You're wondering about that — we're going after lunch."
✅ *Redirect:* "Help me fold these towels?"

Emotion calms the brain. Task changes the focus.

✅ **4. Activities That Keep the Brain Alive**

Alzheimer's patients still benefit from stimulation.

✅ Good activities:

- Folding towels
- Simple puzzles
- Coloring or drawing
- Shelling peas or peeling fruit
- Listening to music
- Looking at photo albums
- Watering plants
- Walking outdoors

These activities:
✅ Reduce depression
✅ Slow memory decline
✅ Improve sleep
✅ Reduce behavior problems

✓5. Managing Eating and Bathing Challenges

✓Eating Problems

Many patients:

- Forget to eat
- Forget how to chew
- Overeat sweets
- Eat unsafe items

✓Solutions:

- Serve finger foods if utensils confuse them
- Keep water visible to prevent dehydration
- Avoid arguing about food — distract instead
- High-calorie snacks if they are losing weight

✓Bathing Problems

Bathing may feel scary:

- Cold water
- Confusion
- Feeling watched
- Hearing echoes

✓Solutions:

- Warm bathroom & towels
- Calm music
- Dim lights
- Let them hold a towel for dignity
- Caregiver of same gender if possible

✅6. Preventing Nighttime Problems

Many Alzheimer's patients get worse in the evening — called **Sundowning**.

✅Reduce naps during the day
✅Keep room dark at night
✅Motion sensor night-lights
✅Avoid caffeine after 2 PM
✅Quiet evenings, no arguments, no loud TV

✅7. Wandering Prevention

Wandering is one of the most dangerous symptoms.

✅GPS bracelet
✅Install door alarms
✅Put "STOP" signs on doors
✅Let them walk outdoors with supervision
✅Leave a recent photo at home for emergencies

✅8. Medications & Medical Care

Doctors may prescribe:

- Memory medications (Donepezil, Memantine)
- Sleep or anxiety medications
- Vitamins (B12, Vitamin D)

Not a cure — but they help slow symptoms.

✅9. Caregiver Mental Health – The Hidden Crisis

Caring for Alzheimer's can destroy a caregiver's health if they are not supported.

Common caregiver problems:

- Depression
- Stress

- Exhaustion
- Social isolation
- Financial strain

✅ **Caregiver Survival Rules**

✅Ask for help — do NOT do everything alone
✅Join support groups
✅Learn the disease
✅Rest and take breaks
✅Seek respite care or adult day centers

Caregivers must protect THEIR health, or both will suffer.

✅ **10. Myths & Pitfalls in Alzheimer's Care**

Mistake Families Make	Why It Hurts
Arguing or correcting	Increases anger & confusion
Leaving the person alone	High risk of accidents or wandering
Assuming they "understand"	They forget quickly, even while nodding
Not preparing legal/medical documents early	Too late to sign once memory is worse
Thinking diet or vitamins will cure it	No cure — only symptom management

✅ **Pro Tips (That Professionals Use)**

✅Play the person's favorite music during meals → increases appetite
✅Let them "help" with chores → gives confidence and purpose
✅Use soft lighting → reduces agitation
✅Keep noise low → brain becomes overwhelmed easily
✅Never say: "Don't you remember?"

✅ **Simple Visual: Care Strategy Triangle**

```
          SAFETY
      /            \
ROUTINE ---- COMMUNICATION
```

If one side breaks, behavior problems increase.

✅ **Quick Reference Checklist**

✅ Calm voice
✅ Short instructions
✅ No arguing
✅ Daily routine
✅ Safe home
✅ Activities & movement
✅ Hydration
✅ Caregiver rest
✅ Doctor check-ups

✅ **Final Message**

Caring for someone with Alzheimer's is not about trying to "fix" their memory.
It is about giving them **comfort, dignity, safety, and love**.

You cannot change the disease —
but you can change the environment, the communication, and the quality of life.

What Are the Symptoms of Alzheimer's Disease?

Alzheimer's disease does not arrive suddenly. It sneaks in quietly—first stealing short-term memories, then language, judgment, and eventually the ability to walk, swallow, and speak. Most families do not notice the first signs, or they assume "it's just aging." In truth, the symptoms are very specific and follow a predictable pattern.

To understand Alzheimer's symptoms, we'll look at:

1. Early, Middle, and Late-Stage Symptoms
2. Behavior and personality changes
3. Rare but serious symptoms families overlook
4. A real-life story
5. Diagrams and charts
6. Hidden mistakes families make and how to respond

✅A Real Story – *"But He Seems Fine…"*

Jamal, 69, had always been a businessman—organized, confident, brilliant with numbers. His wife noticed he was misplacing bills, repeating questions, and struggling to follow conversations. The family brushed it off:
"He's just tired."
"He's getting older."
"He's stressed."

One afternoon, Jamal got lost driving home from a grocery store he had gone to for 20 years. When the police found him, he couldn't explain where he lived. That moment changed everything. The family realized these weren't small memory slips—this was **Alzheimer's.**

Lesson:
Symptoms are subtle at first. Many families ignore them until something dangerous happens.

✅✅The 10 Major Symptom Categories of Alzheimer's

Alzheimer's is not only "memory loss."
It affects every part of life.

```
THINKING   | MEMORY   | BEHAVIOR | SPEECH |
MOVEMENT | JUDGMENT
```

✓1. Short-Term Memory Loss (Most Famous Symptom)

Memory is the first domino to fall.

Early Signs:

- Asking the same question repeatedly
- Forgetting recent conversations
- Losing items and accusing others of theft
- Missing appointments or events
- Relying heavily on notes or reminders

Why It Happens:

The **hippocampus**, the brain's memory center, is the first area damaged.

```
HEALTHY HIPPOCAMPUS → stores new memories
ALZHEIMER'S HIPPOCAMPUS → cannot record new information
```

This is why a person may remember events from childhood but forget yesterday.

✓2. Difficulty Planning, Problem-Solving, & Logic

Tasks requiring thinking become harder:

- Paying bills
- Balancing a checkbook
- Following a recipe
- Understanding instructions
- Making decisions

Even simple things—like choosing clothes—can create stress.

✅3. Disorientation to Time or Place

A person may:

- Forget what month or year it is
- Get lost in familiar places
- Wander or leave home unexpectedly
- Confuse day and night

Danger sign: A person who suddenly walks outside confused is not "just forgetful."

✅4. Language & Communication Problems

Alzheimer's slowly shuts down language.
This is called **aphasia**.

Symptoms:

- Trouble finding words ("Where is the… the… that thing?")
- Calling objects the wrong name
- Short or incomplete sentences
- Repeating phrases
- Difficulty understanding speech

Later, speech becomes very limited:

- Only a few words
- Echoing others
- Complete silence

✅5. Personality & Behavior Changes

This is the symptom families struggle with most emotionally.
The disease changes **who the person is**.

Common behaviors:

- Irritability
- Depression
- Anxiety
- Suspicion or paranoia
- Crying or sudden anger
- Loss of interest in hobbies
- Restlessness or pacing

Some become aggressive, others quiet and withdrawn. **It is not their fault.** Their brain can no longer regulate emotions.

✅6. Poor Judgment & Unsafe Decisions

This symptom can be dangerous.

Examples:

- Giving away money to strangers
- Not dressing for cold weather
- Leaving the stove on
- Believing scams
- Driving when unsafe

Families often say:
"He used to be smart. Why is he doing this?"
Because Alzheimer's damages the **frontal lobe**, the part of the brain that controls judgment.

✅7. Trouble With Spatial Awareness & Movement

- Difficulty walking

- Poor balance
- Trouble sitting or standing
- Shuffling feet
- Physical rigidity

This happens as Alzheimer's spreads to movement areas of the brain.

✅8. Hallucinations or Delusions *(not in every patient)*

Some people:

- See people who are not there
- Hear voices or sounds
- Think family members are strangers
- Believe someone stole their belongings

This can be frightening, but arguing does not help. Reassurance and redirection is the safest approach.

✅9. Sleep Disturbance & Sundowning

In the late afternoon or evening, many patients become:

- Agitated
- Confused
- Angry
- Restless
- Difficult to control

This is called **Sundowning.**

They may pace, wander, cry, or insist on going "home," even if they are already home.

✅10. Loss of Physical Function (Late Stage)

As the brain shrinks, the body loses control:

- Difficulty swallowing
- Incontinence (bladder and bowel)
- Cannot walk, sit, or hold objects
- Bed-bound
- Frequent infections
- Silent or unable to speak

Alzheimer's eventually affects the brain stem—the system that controls breathing and swallowing. In late stage, many people pass away from pneumonia or infections.

✅Stages of Symptoms: From Mild → Severe

Stage Chart

Stage	Symptoms
Mild (Early)	Forgetfulness, repeating questions, mood changes, losing objects
Moderate (Middle)	Wandering, confusion, sleep problems, aggression, hallucinations, difficulty with daily tasks
Severe (Late)	Can't walk or speak, eating problems, total care needed, no recognition of family

✅Visual Progression Diagram

```
EARLY →    Memory slips → Confusion → Mood
changes
MIDDLE →   Wandering → Hallucinations →
Loss of independence
LATE →     Loss of speech → Loss of
```

mobility → Bedbound

✅Early Warning Signs Families Often Miss

✅Frequently losing keys or wallet
✅Asking the same question repeatedly
✅Taking longer to do familiar tasks
✅Getting overwhelmed by choices
✅Difficulty managing money
✅Unusual anger or sadness
✅Losing interest in hobbies
✅Constantly checking the time
✅Poor hygiene or grooming

Many relatives mistake these for:

- Stress
- Aging
- Laziness
- Depression

But when **multiple** symptoms appear together, Alzheimer's may be starting.

✅The "Memory vs. Aging Test"

Normal Aging	Alzheimer's
Forgets names but remembers later	Forgets names and never recalls
Loses keys sometimes	Hides keys in strange places, can't find them
Needs a reminder	Needs reminders constantly
Makes small mistakes	Dangerous mistakes (stove, driving, money)
Tells a story twice	Repeats same question every 5

Normal Aging	Alzheimer's
	minutes
Aware of the forgetfulness	Denies it, angry or confused

✅ **Hidden Behavior Symptoms Families Rarely Recognize as Alzheimer's**

Families often report:

- "He used to be calm, now he's angry all the time"
- "She follows me room to room"
- "He's up all night pacing"
- "She thinks people are stealing her things"
- "He doesn't want to shower"

These are all **classic Alzheimer's symptoms.**

Why?

Because the brain is losing the ability to:

- reason
- control impulses
- understand reality
- remember conversations

✅ **Why Alzheimer's Patients Get Angry or Aggressive**

Not because they are mean.
Because they are:

- scared
- confused
- overwhelmed

- unable to explain their needs

A person may shout, hit, or push not out of violence, but because language is failing and fear is rising.

✅Why Repetition Happens

When memory disappears, every question feels new.

Example:
You answer:
"When is dinner? In 1 hour."

But 2 minutes later, their brain has erased it.

So they ask again.
And again.
And again.

✅Why Wandering Happens

The person is not "trying to run away."
Common reasons:

- Boredom
- Searching for a familiar place
- Looking for a bathroom
- Seeking someone they remember
- Confused about time or location

✅Pro-Tips for Managing Symptoms

✅**Never ask:** "Don't you remember?"
✅**Avoid arguing or correcting**
✅Keep instructions short
✅Use calm voice and gentle touch
✅Keep routines predictable
✅Remove dangerous items

✅Play calming music in the evening
✅Use night-lights to reduce fear

✅What DOESN'T Work (But Families Often Try)

Ineffective Response	Why it Fails
Arguing	They cannot understand logic
Forcing them to remember	Brain cannot store new information
Yelling or scolding	Increases fear → aggression
Saying "You're wrong"	Triggers humiliation and anxiety
Leaving them alone when upset	Anxiety increases → wandering

✅A Brief Emotional Perspective

Alzheimer's is like waking up in a world where:

- Nothing is familiar
- Faces are strange
- Time is confusing
- Rooms feel wrong
- Everyone corrects you
- Your own mind is disappearing

Understanding this helps caregivers respond with empathy instead of frustration.

✅Summary Chart

```
Alzheimer's Symptoms

COGNITIVE:
- Memory loss
```

```
- Confusion
- Poor judgment
- Speech problems
- Getting lost

BEHAVIORAL:
- Anger, crying
- Hallucinations
- Wandering
- Repeating questions
- Suspicion/paranoia

PHYSICAL:
- Balance problems
- Incontinence
- Difficulty swallowing
- Loss of mobility
```

✅ Final Message

Alzheimer's symptoms are not random.
They follow a pattern, slowly increasing as the brain loses function.

- Memory fades
- Logic weakens
- Behavior changes
- The body shuts down

Recognizing early symptoms gives families a chance to prepare, seek treatment, protect safety, and provide compassionate care.

How Doctors Diagnose Alzheimer's Disease

Why getting the right diagnosis early can change someone's entire future

Most people believe Alzheimer's can only be diagnosed for sure **after a person's memory becomes severely impaired**. But here's the surprising truth:

✅Modern medicine can detect early Alzheimer's **years before symptoms become obvious**,
✅Sometimes even before the patient or family notices memory problems.

Early diagnosis can:

- Slow down cognitive decline
- Help plan care, legal affairs, and medications
- Allow access to treatments and clinical trials
- Reduce stress caused by confusion or mislabeling symptoms

But the diagnosis is **not a single test**—it's a step-by-step medical investigation.

✅A Short, Real Story

Maria, 67, began forgetting small things—keys, doctor dates, repeating stories. Her family assumed it was "normal aging" or stress. She refused to see a doctor, afraid of the word *Alzheimer's*.

Finally, after getting lost driving to her sister's home—a place she'd visited for 30 years—her son convinced her to see a neurologist.

Maria went through memory testing, blood work, and a brain scan. The result: **early Alzheimer's disease**.

BUT here's the twist:

Because she was diagnosed early, doctors started medication, changed her diet, encouraged exercise, and created routines to support memory.

Two years later, Maria is **independent**, able to garden, cook, and enjoy life.
If she waited, she might already need daily supervision.

This is why early diagnosis matters.

✓How Doctors Diagnose Alzheimer's: The 7-Step Process

STEP	WHAT HAPPENS	WHY IT MATTERS
1	Medical History & Interview	Identifies warning signs & past illnesses
2	Physical & Neurological Exam	Rules out other brain or nerve problems
3	Cognitive Testing	Measures memory, language, thinking abilities
4	Blood Tests	Detects treatable causes of memory loss
5	Brain Scans (CT/MRI/PET)	Shows brain shrinkage or abnormal proteins
6	Biomarker Tests	Detect Alzheimer proteins in brain or spinal fluid
7	Monitoring Symptoms Over Time	Confirms progression and stage

✓STEP 1: Medical History & Interview

Doctors ask:

- What symptoms are happening?
- How long have they been happening?
- Is the person forgetting names? Words? Places?
- Do they repeat questions?

- Any personality or mood changes?

Family members are extremely important here—sometimes patients deny symptoms or are unaware of them.

✅ **Common questions doctors ask family**

- Do they forget appointments?
- Do they get lost?
- Do they manage money or bills normally?
- Any sudden anger or confusion?
- Are they locking themselves out?
- Is cooking becoming unsafe?

✅ **STEP 2: Physical & Neurological Exam**

Doctors test:

- Balance
- Vision & eye movements
- Hearing
- Reflexes
- Coordination
- Walking gait

Why?
Because **not all memory loss is Alzheimer's.**

✅ Stroke
✅ Parkinson's
✅ Brain tumor
✅ Vitamin deficiency
✅ Thyroid disease
✅ Depression
can all cause symptoms that look like Alzheimer's.

✅STEP 3: Cognitive & Memory Testing

Doctors use standardized tests:

✅Mini-Mental State Examination (MMSE)

Score out of 30 points.
Tests:

- Orientation (date, place)
- Memory
- Language
- Attention
- Copying shapes

SCORE	INTERPRETATION
25–30	Normal cognition
20–24	Mild dementia
10–19	Moderate dementia
0–9	Severe dementia

✅MoCA (Montreal Cognitive Assessment)

More sensitive, especially in early Alzheimer's.

✅Clock Drawing Test

The patient draws a clock with numbers and a time.

A normal brain:

```
        12
   11         1
10               2
9                 3
8                 4
   7            5
        6
```

A brain with Alzheimer's often:

- Misplaces numbers
- Draws only part of the clock
- Cannot set correct time

✅STEP 4: Blood Tests

Blood tests are not for *detecting* Alzheimer's—they are for eliminating other causes.

Doctors check for:
✅Thyroid problems
✅Vitamin B-12 deficiency
✅Liver + Kidney problems
✅Infections
✅Anemia
✅Inflammation

Fun fact:
A vitamin B-12 deficiency can mimic dementia—and is 100% reversible with treatment.

✅STEP 5: Brain Imaging

✅CT Scan or MRI

Shows:

- Brain shrinkage
- Stroke damage
- Tumors
- Hydrocephalus (fluid buildup)

Typical Alzheimer's pattern:

```
NORMAL BRAIN:   dense, full structure
```

```
ALZHEIMER BRAIN: hippocampus shrinkage,
enlarged ventricles
```

✅ **PET Scan (FDG-PET)**

Measures how active brain cells are.
Alzheimer's brain shows **low activity** in memory areas.

✅ **STEP 6: Biomarker Tests (Most Advanced)**

Biomarkers reveal **Alzheimer proteins**:

- **Amyloid plaques**
- **Tau tangles**

✅ **CSF (Spinal Fluid Test)**

- Detects abnormal amyloid + tau levels
- Very accurate, used in hospitals and research centers

✅ **Amyloid PET Scan**
Shows amyloid deposits in the brain

✅ **Blood Biomarker Tests**
New and becoming more available:

- p-tau217
- p-tau181
  These may soon replace spinal taps.

✅ **The 5 Warning Patterns Doctors Look For**

Brain Function	Early Changes	What Families Notice
Memory	Trouble learning new info	Asking same questions
Language	Trouble finding words	Saying "the thing", "you know…"

Brain Function	Early Changes	What Families Notice
Orientation	Getting lost	Confusing dates/places
Judgment	Poor decisions	Money mistakes, scams
Personality	Mood or behavior shifts	Anger, paranoia, depression

✅Common Misconceptions People Believe

Myth	Truth
"Memory loss is normal aging."	Mild forgetfulness is normal—Alzheimer's causes decline that interferes with daily life.
"You can diagnose it with one scan."	Diagnosis requires a combination of tests.
"Doctors can't know until someone is very sick."	New tests detect early-stage Alzheimer's.
"If symptoms improve one day, it's not Alzheimer's."	Alzheimer's symptoms fluctuate day-to-day.

✅Hidden Pitfalls & Pro Tips

✅Pitfall #1: Waiting too long

Families often delay diagnosis because:

- They hope symptoms are temporary
- They fear the stigma
- The patient refuses to go

⛔But waiting can cause:

- Unsafe driving
- Financial exploitation

- Wandering
- Medication mistakes

✅ **Pro-tip:** If you notice changes, keep a **symptom diary**:

- What happened?
- When?
- How often?
- Who noticed it?

Doctors take this very seriously.

✅ Pitfall #2: Believing memory tests are pointless

Some people argue:
"My parent remembers birthdays—so they're fine."

But Alzheimer's doesn't start with old memories.
It starts with **new memories**.

That's why the question:
"What did you eat for breakfast?"
is more important than
"What was your wedding year?"

✅ Pitfall #3: Only seeing a general doctor

General physicians are helpful—but a **neurologist** or **geriatric specialist** gives deeper evaluation.

✅ Best experts:

- Neurologist
- Neuropsychologist
- Geriatrician
- Memory clinic

✅Pitfall #4: Thinking no treatment exists

While Alzheimer's is not curable, early diagnosis allows:

- Medications to slow decline
- Better safety planning
- Lifestyle changes that protect the brain
- Emotional preparation
- Access to new therapies and research

Without diagnosis, families miss these benefits.

✅Do Diagnosis Methods Actually Work?

Yes—but no single method is perfect. Together, they create a full picture.

METHOD	Detects Alzheimer Early	Detects Other Causes	Cost
Memory tests	✅Yes	❌No	Low
CT/MRI	✅Moderate	✅Yes	Medium
PET scan	✅Very accurate	❌Not for other causes	High
Blood tests	✅Emerging accuracy	✅Yes	Medium
Spinal tap (CSF)	✅Highly accurate	✅Yes	Medium–High

Most accurate diagnosis = **PET scan + CSF biomarkers + cognitive testing**
(Used in advanced hospitals and research centers)

✅Where Diagnosis Is Heading — The Future

Within the next 5–10 years:
✅Blood tests may diagnose Alzheimer before symptoms

✅Treatments may start even earlier
✅Prevention-based medicine may become standard

This means today's patients benefit from breakthroughs tomorrow.

✅Summary Chart

```
HOW DOCTORS DIAGNOSE ALZHEIMER'S?

1. Patient Interview + Family History
2. Memory and Cognitive Tests
3. Blood Tests (rule out other problems)
4. Brain Scan (MRI/CT/PET)
5. Biomarker Tests (CSF / blood)
6. Long-term monitoring
```

Diagnosis is like assembling a puzzle—each test adds a piece.

✅Final Message

If you suspect changes in yourself or someone you love:

✅Early diagnosis = more independence
✅Early diagnosis = stronger treatment effect
✅Early diagnosis = safer, happier life

Alzheimer's is not just a memory disease.
It is a brain disease—and the earlier we find it, the better we fight it.

How to Prevent Early Alzheimer?

Science-backed strategies to protect the brain before symptoms appear

For decades, people believed Alzheimer's was something that "just happens with age."
But modern neuroscience discovered something shocking:

✅Alzheimer's can begin **20 years before the first memory problem**
✅Brain cells start changing long before symptoms
✅Lifestyle and habits can delay — or speed up — brain aging

That means prevention isn't just possible…
It can be life-changing.

✅A Short Relatable Story

Kevin, age 45, worked long hours, slept late, ate fast food, and rarely exercised. His father died with Alzheimer's at 70, so he knew the risk was real — but he ignored it.
Memory problems started earlier than he expected: forgotten appointments, difficulty concentrating, mixing up client information. He thought it was stress.

After speaking to a neurologist, Kevin discovered he had:

- Vitamin D deficiency
- High blood sugar
- High inflammation markers
- Poor sleep quality
- Very high processed food intake

He changed:
✅Daily walking
✅Earlier sleep
✅Mediterranean diet

✅Brain exercises
✅Better stress control

One year later, his memory returned to normal, brain fog disappeared, and his risk dramatically decreased.

? Prevention doesn't require perfection — it requires consistency.

✅Why Early Prevention Matters

Most people think Alzheimer's strikes at age 70+.
But the brain changes start decades earlier.

✅Brain Decline Timeline

```
Age 20-40: Brain builds, learns,
strengthens
Age 40-60: First signs of slow shrinkage,
inflammation
Age 60+: Symptoms appear if the brain has
been unprotected
```

That's why **prevention must start early**, especially between **40–60**.

✅Top Proven Strategies to Prevent Early Alzheimer

These are not guesses — they are supported by research from:
✅Harvard
✅Mayo Clinic
✅Cleveland Clinic
✅Alzheimer's Association
✅World Health Organization

We'll cover:

1. Brain-boosting foods (anti-inflammatory, memory protecting)

2. Exercise (the #1 most powerful prevention tool)
3. Sleep protection
4. Brain training and mental stimulation
5. Stress reduction
6. Control of blood pressure & blood sugar
7. Social engagement
8. Avoiding major risk factors
9. Vitamins & supplements backed by science

✅1. Nutrition — Feed the Brain Right

The brain consumes **20–25% of the body's energy**. What you eat literally changes how your brain functions.

✅Best Diets for Brain Protection

Diet	Effect
MIND Diet	Specifically designed to reduce Alzheimer's risk
Mediterranean Diet	Reduces inflammation & protects blood vessels
DASH Diet	Controls blood pressure (big Alzheimer risk factor)

People who strictly follow the **MIND diet** have up to:
✅**53% lower risk** of Alzheimer's
Even moderate followers have:
✅**35% lower risk**

✅Brain-Smart Foods

✅Omega-3 foods: salmon, sardines, walnuts, chia, flax
✅Berries: blueberries, blackberries, strawberries
✅Leafy greens: spinach, kale, arugula

✅Olive oil instead of vegetable oil
✅Whole grains instead of refined flour
✅Turmeric + black pepper (anti-inflammatory)
✅Green tea & dark chocolate (antioxidants)

Foods that Accelerate Alzheimer's

Avoid or Reduce	Why
Processed sugar	Creates inflammation & memory decline
Trans fats (margarine, fried snacks)	Damages blood vessels in brain
Processed meats	Increases inflammation
Soda & energy drinks	Linked to brain shrinking
Excess alcohol	Kills neurons

✅2. Movement — The #1 Brain Protector

Exercise is more powerful than any pill.

It:
✅Increases blood flow to the brain
✅Grows new brain cells in the hippocampus
✅Improves memory and mood

✅Best Types of Exercise

Type	Benefits
Walking 30 min/day	Reduces dementia risk up to 40%
Strength training	Protects neurons & balance
Aerobic exercise	Best for blood flow + oxygen
Dancing	Memory, coordination, social connection

? **Scientific insight**:

Every time your heart beats faster, **your brain gets more oxygen**.
That oxygen grows new neural connections.

✅3. Sleep — Memory's Filtration System

When we sleep, the brain **cleans toxins**, especially **amyloid**, the protein responsible for Alzheimer's plaques.

If you sleep less than **6 hours per night**, your brain can't remove waste.

✅Sleep Checklist

✅7–9 hours nightly
✅No screens 30–60 minutes before bed
✅Avoid heavy meals late at night
✅Keep a cool, dark room
✅Limit caffeine after 2 PM

? **Hidden pitfall:**
People who snore loudly or stop breathing during the night may have **sleep apnea**, which increases Alzheimer's risk.
Treatment can dramatically help memory.

✅4. Mental Activity — The Brain Loves Challenges

The brain is like a muscle:
If you don't use it, you lose it.

✅Brain-building activities

- Learn a new language
- Play strategy games
- Play music or learn an instrument
- Solve puzzles or crosswords
- Read every day

- Teach or tutor someone else
- Take new classes

Brain imaging studies show:
People who remain mentally active have **thicker, healthier cortex** and **slower memory decline**.

✅5. Social Interaction — Humans Keep Each Other Alive

Isolation increases Alzheimer's risk as much as **smoking** does.

When you talk, think, laugh, and share ideas:
✅Your brain forms new connections
✅Mood improves
✅Memory improves

✅**Stay socially connected:**

- Join clubs
- Visit family or neighbors
- Volunteer
- Attend religious or community events
- Video call relatives

A **lonely brain declines faster**.

✅6. Manage Blood Pressure & Blood Sugar

Here's a surprising fact most people don't know:

✅Alzheimer's is connected to heart and metabolic health.
Some scientists even call it **"Type 3 Diabetes."**

✅**High Blood Pressure damages:**

- Brain blood vessels
- Memory areas

- Thinking speed

✅**High Blood Sugar:**

- Causes inflammation
- Damages neurons
- Increases amyloid plaques

✅Healthy target numbers:

- Blood pressure: 120/80
- Fasting sugar: 70–100 mg/dL
- A1C: below 5.7%

✅**7. Stress Management**

Chronic stress releases cortisol, which **shrinks the hippocampus** — the center of memory.

✅Best anti-stress habits:

- Meditation
- Prayer
- Deep breathing
- Yoga or stretching
- Gardening
- Spending time outdoors
- Listening to calming music

Even **10 minutes per day** changes brain chemistry.

✅8. Avoid Major Brain Risks

Risk Factor	Why it matters
Smoking	Damages blood flow & brain oxygen
Heavy alcohol use	Kills neurons
Head injuries	Increase risk of early dementia
Sitting too much	Reduces blood flow & memory
Untreated depression	Memory areas shrink

✅Wear helmets
✅Quit smoking
✅Limit alcohol
✅Be physically active

✅9. Vitamins & Supplements That Help

Not magic pills — but helpful if there are deficiencies.

✅Vitamin B-12
✅Vitamin D
✅Omega-3 fish oil
✅Curcumin (turmeric extract)
✅Magnesium
✅Green tea extract

Always check with a doctor first — especially for seniors.

✓Brain-Protective Diagram

```
THE BRAIN HEALTH PYRAMID

              | Sleep |
              |_______|
          | Nutrition |
          |___________|
      | Movement & Exercise |
      |_____________________|
| Stress Control & Mental Activity |
|__________________________________|
             LIFESTYLE
```

Everything works together.
Skipping one weakens all.

✓Common Myths

Myth	Reality
Alzheimer's is genetic — nothing you can do.	90% of cases are NOT purely genetic. Lifestyle matters.
Brain games are enough.	Only one part. Exercise + diet + sleep are stronger.
If you forget things, you already have Alzheimer's.	Stress, vitamin deficiency, depression can also cause memory issues.
You must be old to worry about it.	Prevention works best between ages 40–60.

✓A Clear, Simple Action Plan

✓DAILY

- Walk 30 minutes
- Eat berries, leafy greens, olive oil

- Avoid processed sugar
- Sleep 7–9 hours
- Talk to at least 1 person
- Learn or practice something new

✅ **WEEKLY**

- Strength training 2–3 times
- Omega–3 foods
- Social gatherings
- Meditation or yoga

✅ **YEARLY**

- Check blood pressure, sugar, B-12, vitamin D
- Cognitive baseline test after age 55

✅ **Final Message**

You can't change your age.
You can't change your genes.

But you CAN change:
✅ What you eat
✅ How you move
✅ How you sleep
✅ How you think
✅ How you manage stress

And these changes can **delay Alzheimer's for years**, or in some people, **prevent it completely**.

A healthy brain is not luck —
It is a lifestyle.

Simple habits that protect the brain without medication

Alzheimer's is not an overnight illness — it develops silently for years.
The good news?

Up to 40% of Alzheimer's cases can be prevented or delayed using natural lifestyle strategies backed by science.

Most people believe prevention is complicated.
But the brain is surprisingly responsive to simple daily actions:

- Movement
- Food
- Social interaction
- Sleep
- Mental stimulation
- Stress control

The natural approach is not "alternative medicine"—
it is **evidence-based neuroscience**.

✅A Short, Relatable Story

Linda, 61, noticed she was forgetting small things:
losing keys, repeating conversations, forgetting common words.

Her mother had Alzheimer's.
Her grandmother had Alzheimer's.

Linda assumed it was destiny.

One memory specialist told her:

> "Genes load the gun — lifestyle pulls the trigger."

So she changed:

✅ Switched to olive oil instead of butter
✅ Walked every morning
✅ Did puzzles and online memory games
✅ Reduced sugar and processed food
✅ Slept earlier and deeper
✅ Started volunteering

Within 6 months:

- Her memory improved
- Her mood stabilized
- Her energy increased
- Her confidence returned

She didn't need extreme diets, expensive supplements, or medical procedures.
She needed habits.

This is the power of natural prevention.

✅✅Natural Alzheimer Prevention Strategies Backed By Science

✅1. Eat Foods That Repair the Brain

The brain is made of:

- 60% fat
- 25% cholesterol
- Millions of neurons that depend on nutrients

Natural, anti-inflammatory foods protect brain cells and help them communicate.

✓The MIND Diet — the #1 proven "brain diet"

Category	Eat Frequently	Why it Works
Leafy greens	Spinach, kale, arugula, chard	Prevent brain aging
Berries	Blueberries, blackberries, strawberries	Reduce oxidative damage
Healthy oils	Olive oil, avocado oil	Prevent artery damage
Whole grains	Oats, brown rice, quinoa	Stable energy to brain
Fish	Salmon, sardines, tuna	Omega-3 strengthens neurons
Nuts & Seeds	Walnuts, almonds, flax, chia	Build brain cell membranes

✓Foods that *damage* the brain

Avoid or Limit	Why
Deep fried foods	Create inflammatory chemicals
Processed sugar	Shrinks memory centers
Margarine & trans fats	Block blood flow to brain
Soda & energy drinks	Increase insulin resistance
Highly processed snacks	High in chemicals & preservatives

✓2. Exercise: Natural Medicine for the Brain

You don't need gyms or trainers.
Walking alone can change the brain.

✓Why exercise works

- Grows **new neurons** in the hippocampus

- Increases **blood flow and oxygen**
- Improves **learning and concentration**
- Lowers **inflammation**
- Boosts **mood and motivation**

✅ **Best natural exercises**

Activity	Brain Benefit
Walking	40% reduced dementia risk
Dancing	Coordination + memory + joy
Swimming	High oxygen to brain
Cycling	Cardiovascular strength
Tai chi / yoga	Balance + calm + focus

Fun fact:
The hippocampus (memory center) can actually **increase size** in adults who exercise regularly.

✅ **3. Sleep: The Brain's Cleaning System**

During sleep, the brain washes out toxic proteins, including **amyloid**, the Alzheimer's protein.

If you sleep <6 hours consistently:

- toxins accumulate
- brain cells weaken
- memory declines faster

✅ **Natural sleep improvement tips**

✅ Go to bed at the same time daily
✅ Eliminate screens 1 hour before bed
✅ Drink chamomile or warm milk
✅ Dark, cool bedroom
✅ Avoid caffeine after the afternoon

✅Read or stretch before bed

Major pitfall: Loud snoring + daytime fatigue = possible sleep apnea
Treating it can improve memory instantly.

✅4. Brain Stimulation — Use It or Lose It

The brain needs challenges.
When you learn something new, your neurons build **new pathways**.

✅Natural brain exercises

✅Reading
✅Learning a language
✅Playing chess or strategy games
✅Memorizing poems or scriptures
✅Teaching others
✅Learning music
✅Cooking new recipes

Watching TV does **not** count — the brain is passive.

✅5. Natural Stress Control

Chronic stress releases **cortisol**, which damages memory areas.

You don't need pills.
You need habits that calm the nervous system naturally.

✅Natural stress relievers

✅Meditation
✅Prayer
✅Walking in nature
✅Deep breathing
✅Gardening
✅Journaling

✅ Spending time with pets
✅ Listening to calming music

? People who meditate regularly show:

- Larger memory centers
- Better attention
- Lower inflammation

✅ 6. Social Interaction — Invisible Brain Medicine

Humans are made for connection.
Loneliness increases dementia risk as much as smoking.

Talking, laughing, and sharing stories stimulates:

- Language centers
- Memory networks
- Emotional processing

✅ Natural ways to stay socially active

✅ Visit relatives
✅ Join a club or community group
✅ Attend religious services
✅ Volunteer
✅ Cook or walk with a neighbor
✅ Take classes with others

A connected brain is a stronger brain.

✅ 7. Protect the Brain from Physical Damage

Natural but critical:

✅ Wear seatbelts
✅ Wear helmets during cycling or motorbiking
✅ Prevent falls at home
✅ Manage blood pressure

✅Quit smoking
✅Limit alcohol

One major head injury doubles dementia risk.

✅8. Control Blood Sugar & Blood Pressure Naturally

Alzheimer's is strongly linked with:

- diabetes
- high blood pressure
- obesity

Natural ways to control them:

✅Cut sugary drinks
✅Eat whole foods
✅Walk after meals
✅Drink enough water
✅Eat smaller portions
✅Increase fiber intake

✅10 minutes of walking after meals reduces blood sugar naturally.

✅9. Natural Herbs & Supplements (Scientifically Studied)

Not miracle cures — but helpful with doctor approval:

✅**Turmeric (curcumin)**
Reduces inflammation, crosses blood-brain barrier

✅**Omega-3 fish oil**
Strengthens brain cells, improves memory

✅**Vitamin D**
Low levels linked with dementia

✅**Vitamin B-12**
Deficiency causes severe memory problems

✅ **Magnesium**
Supports brain relaxation and sleep

✅ **Green tea extract**
Powerful antioxidants

⛔ Avoid unproven pills advertised as "memory boosters." Most don't work and waste money.

✅ **Simple Natural Prevention Pyramid**

```
        DAILY HABITS
  Sleep   Exercise   Nutrition
_______________________________
 Mental Activity  Social Life
_______________________________
 Stress Control & Healthy Blood
          LIFESTYLE
```

✅ **Common Myths About Natural Prevention**

Myth	Reality
"If Alzheimer's runs in my family, I can't prevent it."	Lifestyle can reduce risk by **40–60%**, even with family history.
"Brain games alone prevent dementia."	Only one part — exercise and diet are stronger.
"Herbs can cure Alzheimer's."	Herbs support health, but no natural cure exists.
"You must start when you are old."	Prevention works best **before** symptoms — ages 40–60.

✅ **Hidden Pitfalls**

❌ Drinking juice instead of eating whole fruit
(juice spikes sugar, no fiber)

❌ Sitting for long hours
(even if you exercise later, long sitting weakens brain

circulation)

✅Fix: Stand or walk every hour

❌Multitasking on screens
(reduces attention span and short-term memory)

✅Fix: Single-tasking improves focus

✅**A Simple 30-Day Natural Prevention Plan**

✅**DAILY**

- 30-minute walk
- 7–9 hours sleep
- Leafy greens + olive oil
- No sugary drinks
- Social interaction
- 10 minutes of brain training
- 10 minutes of stress relief

✅**WEEKLY**

- Fish 2–3 times
- Strength training twice
- Volunteer or group activity
- New learning (class, hobby)

✅**MONTHLY**

- Check blood pressure at home
- Track weight and sleep habits

Natural prevention is **not a diet** — it is a lifestyle.

✅ Final Message

You don't need expensive treatments.
You don't need perfect discipline.
You don't need a scientist to live brain-healthy.

You need simple, natural habits repeated daily.

- Move your body
- Feed your brain
- Sleep deeply
- Stay curious
- Stay connected
- Protect your heart
- Reduce stress

These habits **literally change your brain chemistry**, stop inflammation, and protect memory.

Alzheimer's is not only a disease of age —
it is a disease of lifestyle.
And lifestyle is something we control.

What's the Difference Between Alzheimer's & Dementia?

Most people use the words **"Alzheimer's"** and **"dementia"** as if they are the same. Even many families caring for a loved one will say, *"My mother has dementia—so she has Alzheimer's, right?"*
But here's the truth:

! Dementia is NOT a disease. Alzheimer's IS.
! Dementia is a **general term**—Alzheimer's is just **one specific type.**
! Not all dementia is Alzheimer's—and not all memory

problems are dementia.

This misunderstanding causes major problems: misdiagnosis, wrong treatment paths, and delayed care.
So let's break it down in a way that is simple, visual, and unforgettable.

✅The Quick Difference

Term	What It Means	Key Clue
Dementia	An umbrella term for symptoms that affect memory, reasoning, and daily functioning	A *syndrome* (collection of symptoms), not one disease
Alzheimer's	A specific disease that causes 60–80% of dementia cases	Progressive brain damage from abnormal protein buildup

Think of dementia like saying "fever," and Alzheimer's like influenza.
Many things can cause a fever—just like many conditions can cause dementia.

✅A Visual Breakdown

```
ALL DEMENTIA
  ├── Alzheimer's disease (60-80%)
  ├── Vascular dementia (10-20%)
  ├── Lewy body dementia (5-10%)
  ├── Frontotemporal dementia (2-5%)
  └── Others (Parkinson's dementia, head
trauma-related, etc.)
```

This means:
✔ Someone can have dementia that **is not** Alzheimer's
✔ Someone can have **both** Alzheimer's and vascular changes
✔ Treatment and progression can differ depending on the type

✅ Short Story: The Misdiagnosis Problem

Samuel's daughter thought he had Alzheimer's.
He was forgetting words, losing track of days, and struggling with planning meals. The family started preparing emotionally for an Alzheimer's diagnosis.

But after a brain scan and neurological exam, doctors found something different:

➡ Samuel had **vascular dementia** caused by tiny strokes.
➡ Alzheimer's medication wouldn't have helped.
➡ What DID help? Blood pressure control, exercise, and stroke-prevention treatment.

Within 8 months, his decline slowed dramatically.

✅ The lesson: **Getting the diagnosis right matters.**
Each type needs **different treatments** and has a **different outcome**.

✅ So What Exactly Is Dementia?

✔ A "Syndrome," Not a Disease

Dementia is a set of symptoms caused by brain damage severe enough to affect daily life:

Core symptoms of dementia:

- Memory loss
- Trouble with reasoning or planning
- Difficulty communicating
- Confusion about time or place
- Behavior or personality changes
- Difficulty doing daily tasks

You can have dementia from:

- Alzheimer's disease
- Stroke or blocked blood vessels
- Parkinson's disease
- Lewy body buildup
- Frontotemporal damage
- Repeated head injuries
- Alcohol abuse
- Vitamin deficiency
- Thyroid disorders

➡ Some types of dementia **are treatable or partially reversible**, which is why diagnosis is critical.

✅ So What Makes Alzheimer's Different?

Alzheimer's is a **specific brain disease** where two proteins—**amyloid plaques** and **tau tangles**—build up and kill brain cells.

Symptoms of Alzheimer's

- Memory loss that keeps worsening
- Trouble learning new information
- Getting lost, even in familiar places
- Confusion and word-finding problems
- Personality changes
- Decline in reasoning and judgment

It progresses slowly and is irreversible.

✅Let's Compare: Alzheimer's vs. Other Dementias

Feature	Alzheimer's	Vascular Dementia	Lewy Body Dementia	Frontotemporal Dementia
Main cause	Protein buildup in brain	Stroke or blood flow issues	Abnormal Lewy protein	Damage to frontal/temporal lobes
Early signs	Memory loss	Problem-solving issues	Hallucinations, vivid dreams	Personality/behavior changes
Common ages	65+	60+	50+	45–65
Reversible?	No	Sometimes slowed	No	No
Progression	Slow, steady	Step-by-step decline	Fluctuating	Faster in behavior changes

✅A Diagram to Remember

Why Alzheimer's Is the Most Common Cause of Dementia

```
Total Dementia Cases (100%)
  ├── 60-80% = Alzheimer's
  ├── 10-20% = Vascular
  ├── 5-10% = Lewy Body
  ├── 2-5% = Frontotemporal
  └── <5% = Other causes
```

✔This explains why people confuse them—**most dementia IS Alzheimer's**, but not all.

✅ Big Myth-Busters

❌ Myth #1: "Dementia is normal aging."

✅ **No.** Aging slows memory slightly, but dementia destroys the ability to live independently.

❌ Myth #2: "Memory loss means Alzheimer's."

✅ Memory problems can come from stress, medications, depression, thyroid issues, or vitamin B12 deficiency.

❌ Myth #3: "Alzheimer's only affects seniors."

✅ 5–10% of cases are **early-onset**, appearing in the 40s or 50s.

❌ Myth #4: "All dementia is permanent."

✅ Dementia from:

- vitamin deficiency
- medications
- dehydration
- thyroid problems
  can be improved or reversed

✅ Hidden Pitfall: Misdiagnosis

One of the biggest dangers is assuming **every forgetful person has Alzheimer's.**

Studies show:

- **15–20% of dementia diagnoses are incorrect**
- **Up to 30%** of people labeled with Alzheimer's actually have **mixed dementia**
- Some treatable conditions cause dementia-like symptoms

? This is why doctors use:

- Brain imaging
- Blood tests
- Cognitive testing
- Medical history
- Neurological exams

Accurate diagnosis means **better treatment and better outcomes.**

✅So What Symptoms Suggest Alzheimer's vs Other Dementias?

✅Alzheimer's Early Red Flags

- Memory loss that disrupts daily life
- Repeating the same questions
- Misplacing items and not remembering where
- Trouble planning or problem-solving
- Gradual, steady progression

✅Signs It May NOT Be Alzheimer's

- **Sudden** changes after a stroke → Vascular dementia
- Hallucinations early in disease → Lewy body dementia
- Major personality change first → Frontotemporal dementia
- Shaking and movement problems → Parkinson's dementia

✅Why the Difference Matters for Treatment

Because each dementia type responds differently:

Type	Memory Medications Help?	Lifestyle Treatment?
Alzheimer's	✅Can slow symptoms in early stages	✅Very helpful
Vascular dementia	❌Not very effective	✅Controlling blood pressure, diet, exercise
Lewy body dementia	⚠Some Alzheimer's drugs help memory, but certain antipsychotics can be dangerous	✅Sleep and behavior management
Frontotemporal dementia	❌Alzheimer's drugs don't help	✅Behavior therapies and structure

Imagine giving Alzheimer's drugs to someone with frontal dementia—it won't work, and time is wasted.

✅Real-Life Example: Why Diagnosis Matters

Two patients, same age, both forgetting things:

Patient A	Patient B
Gradual memory decline over 3 years	Decline after a stroke last year
Trouble remembering names	Trouble planning meals, paying bills
Brain scan shows plaques	Brain scan shows vessel damage

➡Patient A = Alzheimer's → Memory medications + cognitive therapy

➡Patient B = Vascular dementia → Blood pressure control + stroke prevention

Both need different care paths.
One size DOES NOT fit all.

✅ Pro Tips for Families

✔ **Get a proper medical diagnosis**—not just "He's forgetting things."
✔ Ask doctors to explain **what type** of dementia it is.
✔ Request:

- Brain imaging
- Blood tests
- Cognitive screening
  ✔ Track changes—sudden change suggests vascular, not Alzheimer's.
  ✔ Don't assume every symptom is memory-related—many affect behavior and judgment first.

✅ The Most Interesting Misunderstood Fact

Many people believe Alzheimer's begins **when symptoms appear.**
But science shows:

? **Alzheimer's can begin 15–20 years before symptoms**
Protein buildup starts silently.
That means lifestyle changes **now** can protect the brain later.

This is why prevention matters—even if no one in your family has the disease.

✅ A Simple Metaphor to Remember

Dementia is a "broken car."
Alzheimer's is **one reason** the engine fails…
but the engine could also break because of:

- no fuel (vitamin deficiency)

- damaged wires (stroke)
- faulty parts (Parkinson's, Lewy body)
- lack of oil (brain inflammation)

Fixing the car **requires knowing what's broken.**

✅ **Conclusion: The Honest, Clear Distinction**

Question	Dementia	Alzheimer's
Is it a disease?	No	Yes
Is it reversible?	Sometimes	No
Does it always worsen?	Usually, but depends on cause	Always
What does it describe?	Decline affecting daily life	Most common cause of dementia

So remember:

✅ **Alzheimer's is the leading cause of dementia, but not the only one.**
✅ **Dementia is a symptom group, not a disease.**
✅ **Correct diagnosis = better treatment, more quality life, fewer mistakes.**

What Causes Dementia?

Most people think dementia is caused only by aging or Alzheimer's.
That's a dangerous misunderstanding.

✅ **Dementia is not caused by aging alone.**
✅ **Dementia is not only Alzheimer's.**
✅ **Dementia is a result of brain cell damage—and there are many ways that damage happens.**

Some causes are permanent.
Some are **preventable.**
Some are even **reversible.**

To protect the brain, we need to understand the root causes—not just the symptoms.

✅First, What Is Dementia Really Caused By?

Dementia occurs when **brain cells are damaged** and can no longer communicate with each other.
This leads to memory loss, confusion, personality changes, and trouble with daily life.

That brain damage can come from:

✔ **Proteins building up in the brain**
✔ **Poor blood flow or strokes**
✔ **Degeneration of the frontal and temporal lobes**
✔ **Trauma**, infections, toxins
✔ **Deficiencies and metabolic disorders**

In short: **dementia is a result, not a single disease.**

✅The 10 Most Common Causes of Dementia

Cause	How It Damages the Brain	Examples
1. Alzheimer's disease	Protein buildup kills brain cells	60–80% of cases
2. Vascular dementia	Strokes/blockages reduce blood flow	Stroke, high BP
3. Lewy body dementia	Abnormal Lewy proteins disrupt signals	Hallucinations
4. Frontotemporal dementia	Degeneration of frontal/temporal lobes	Personality changes
5. Parkinson's disease	Spread of abnormal proteins	Movement + memory decline
6. Chronic alcohol abuse	Shrinks and destroys brain tissue	Wernicke-Korsakoff

Cause	How It Damages the Brain	Examples
7. Repeated brain injury	Trauma damages neurons	Sports injuries, falls
8. Infections	Inflammation damages neurons	HIV, syphilis, meningitis
9. Vitamin/thyroid deficiencies	Brain can't function properly	B12, thyroid disorders
10. Toxic exposure	Heavy metals, drugs, chemicals	Mercury, solvents

✅Notice: **Not all of these are permanent.**
Some can be **treated**, slowed, or reversed.

✅**A Visual Overview**

```
CAUSES OF DEMENTIA
 ├─ Alzheimer's (protein buildup)
 ├─ Vascular (blood flow problems)
 ├─ Lewy Body (abnormal proteins)
 ├─ Frontotemporal (lobe degeneration)
 ├─ Parkinson's
 ├─ Alcohol-related
 ├─ Head trauma
 ├─ Infections
 ├─ Deficiencies
 └─ Toxins
```

Think of dementia like a fire alarm:
? The alarm means there's smoke
? But you need to find **what caused the fire** to fix it.

✅**Cause #1: Alzheimer's Disease (Most Common)**

About **6 in 10** dementia cases are Alzheimer's.
The brain fills with **amyloid plaques** and **tau tangles**, which

choke and destroy brain cells.

Symptoms:

- Memory loss
- Confusion
- Trouble learning
- Personality changes
- Progressive decline

✅Irreversible, but early treatment slows decline in many people.

✅**Cause #2: Vascular Dementia (Blood Flow Problems)**

When the brain doesn't get enough blood, cells die.

This happens due to:

- Stroke
- High blood pressure
- Cholesterol buildup
- Diabetes
- Heart disease

? *Think of it like clogged plumbing: the brain can't get oxygen or nutrients.*

Symptoms:

- Slow thinking
- Planning/organization problems
- Sudden changes after stroke

✅Important: **This type can be prevented or slowed** by controlling blood pressure, diet, and exercise.

✅Cause #3: Lewy Body Dementia

Caused by a buildup of **Lewy proteins**, which disrupt brain chemicals.

Symptoms:

- Visual hallucinations
- Fluctuating attention
- Stiffness or slow movement
- Acting out dreams

⚠Big pitfall: Some medications (antipsychotics) can be dangerous for these patients.

✅Cause #4: Frontotemporal Dementia

Not memory loss first—**personality and behavior change first.**

The frontal and temporal lobes shrink.

Symptoms:

- Impulsive behavior
- Loss of empathy
- Inappropriate actions
- Language difficulty

Often appears earlier—between **45–65 years old**.

✅Cause #5: Parkinson's Disease

Parkinson's can spread from movement areas into memory areas of the brain.

Symptoms:

- Tremors
- Slow movement

- Later memory decline
- Visual and judgment issues

✅**Cause #6: Chronic Alcohol Misuse (Alcohol-Related Dementia)**

Alcohol slowly destroys brain cells and shrinks brain tissue.

Symptoms:

- Poor memory
- Balance issues
- Confusion
- Personality changes

✅Unlike Alzheimer's, alcohol-related dementia **can improve** if drinking stops and nutrition is restored, especially **Vitamin B1 (thiamine)**.

✅**Cause #7: Repeated Head Trauma**

Seen in:

- Boxers
- Football players
- Military veterans
- Accident victims

The brain gets injured repeatedly, leading to **Chronic Traumatic Encephalopathy (CTE)**.

Symptoms:

- Anger
- Impulsive behavior
- Poor judgment

- Memory decline

✅**Cause #8: Infections**

Some infections inflame or directly damage the brain:

- HIV
- Syphilis
- Lyme disease
- Meningitis
- Creutzfeldt-Jakob disease

✅Treating the infection early can **stop the dementia from worsening**.

✅**Cause #9: Vitamin & Thyroid Deficiency (Reversible Dementias)**

Low Vitamin B12, folate, or thyroid hormone mimics dementia.

Symptoms:

- Memory problems
- Fatigue
- Slow thinking
- Confusion

✅With treatment, brain function often improves.
This is why blood tests are essential during diagnosis.

✅**Cause #10: Toxins & Medications**

Some drugs and chemicals permanently damage brain cells:

- Heavy metals (lead, mercury)
- Solvents

- Anesthesia complications
- Drug reactions
- Long-term sedatives

✅Removing the toxin may stop further decline.

✅A Story: The Dementia That Wasn't

Maria, age 67, started forgetting conversations and losing her keys.
Her family feared Alzheimer's and prepared for the worst.

But doctors discovered:
✔ She was extremely low in **Vitamin B12**
✔ She was depressed
✔ Medication side effects were worsening her confusion

After treatment:
✅Her memory returned
✅The "dementia" disappeared

This happens more often than people think.

✅Hidden Pitfall: Misdiagnosis

Experts report:

- **Up to 20%** of dementia cases are actually from treatable causes
- **30% of Alzheimer's diagnoses** are mistaken—patients have "mixed dementia," vascular + Alzheimer's
- Many people labeled with dementia never had proper brain imaging or blood testing

? **Never accept a diagnosis of dementia without testing.**

Required tests should include:

- Blood work (B12, thyroid, infections)

- MRI or CT scan
- Neurological exam
- Medication review
- Cognitive testing

✅ **Myth-Busting**

❌ **Myth: "Dementia is just old age."**

✔ Normal aging = slower recall
✔ Dementia = loss of daily function

❌ **Myth: "Nothing can be done."**

✔ Many causes are preventable
✔ Some are reversible
✔ Early treatment delays decline

❌ **Myth: "Memory loss always means Alzheimer's."**

✔ Dementia can start with **behavior**, **judgment**, or **planning** problems instead.

✅ **Why Knowing the Cause Matters**

Because each cause has different treatment:

Cause	Can Medication Help?	Can It Be Reversed?	Focus of Treatment
Alzheimer's	Sometimes slow symptoms	No	Memory meds, routines
Vascular	Limited	**Sometimes**	Blood pressure, stroke prevention
Lewy Body	Yes for memory, careful with	No	Behavior and sleep

Cause	Can Medication Help?	Can It Be Reversed?	Focus of Treatment
	others		
Frontotemporal	No	No	Therapy, structure
Alcohol-related	Not meds	**Often yes**	Stop alcohol, thiamine
Deficiencies	Not meds	**Yes**	Vitamin/thyroid treatment
Infections	Not meds	**Sometimes yes**	Treat infection

Correct diagnosis = better outcomes.

✅ Pro Tips for Families

✔ If symptoms appear suddenly → check stroke or infection
✔ If personality changes first → consider frontotemporal
✔ If hallucinations begin early → suspect Lewy body
✔ If drinking history → test for alcohol-related dementia
✔ If young (40s–50s) → don't assume Alzheimer's

✔ Most important:
✅ **Get brain imaging and blood tests**
✅ **Review medications**
✅ **Treat reversible causes early**

✅ Conclusion

Dementia is not one disease.
It is the **final result** of brain cell damage—and that damage can come from many sources.

Some causes are preventable.
Some are reversible.
Some require long-term care.

Understanding the cause is the key to treatment, planning, and hope.

Medical Care for Alzheimer's

When a family first hears the words **"Alzheimer's disease,"** one of the very first questions is:

"Is there a cure?"

Right now, there is **no cure**.
But that does **not** mean nothing can be done.

In fact, medical care can:
✅ slow symptoms
✅ protect independence longer
✅ reduce dangerous behaviors
✅ improve quality of life
✅ reduce caregiver stress
✅ allow families to plan, not panic

Alzheimer's treatment is like managing diabetes or heart disease — you **can't eliminate it**, but you can **control the damage** and **extend functional, meaningful life**.

✅ A Short Story: Why Medical Care Matters

Maria's father, Omar, was diagnosed at 72.
At first, the family refused medication — "It's hopeless," they said.

Within a year, his memory worsened, he forgot familiar places, and became paranoid.

Finally, they visited a memory specialist:

✔ He started memory medications
✔ His sleep and mood were treated
✔ Structured routines were added
✔ Diet and exercise improved

Within 6 months:

✅He was calmer
✅Less confused
✅Not wandering
✅Able to dress and eat independently again

No, the disease didn't stop.
But **his dependence decreased and his dignity returned.**
That is the true goal of care.

✅What Does Medical Care Include?

Medical care for Alzheimer's is **not only pills.**
It is a **full care system**:

Category	Example
Medications	Memory drugs, behavior stabilizers
Therapies	Speech, occupational, cognitive
Lifestyle medicine	Diet, exercise, sleep
Safety planning	Home modifications
Emotional support	Caregiver training, counseling
Legal/financial planning	Power of attorney, advance directives

To treat Alzheimer's correctly, **all pieces must work together.**

✅1. Medications That Help Memory and Thinking

There are **two major medication groups** used in Alzheimer's care:

A. Cholinesterase Inhibitors

They boost acetylcholine — a chemical needed for memory and learning.

Common medications:

- Donepezil (Aricept)

- Rivastigmine (Exelon)
- Galantamine (Razadyne)

✅Help with memory
✅Improve daily activities
✅Reduce confusion
✅Often used in early to mid stages

B. NMDA Receptor Blocker

- Memantine (Namenda)

Helps regulate glutamate to protect brain cells from overstimulation.

✅Useful in moderate to late stages
✅Reduces anxiety and behavior issues

Combined Therapy

Memantine + Donepezil is often used for stronger benefit.

✅2. Newer Alzheimer's Medications (Disease-Modifying)

Recent advances have focused on removing **amyloid plaques**, the harmful proteins in the brain.

✅**Lecanemab**
✅**Donanemab**
✅**Aducanumab**

These medications **remove amyloid** and may slow progression in **early-stage** patients.

⚠Limitations:

- Only for early Alzheimer's
- Require brain scans
- Possible side effects: brain swelling or bleeding

- Very expensive in many countries

These are **not cures**, but they **change the disease, not just symptoms.**

✅3. Medicines for Behavior & Mood

Alzheimer's can cause:

- Aggression
- Depression
- Anxiety
- Hallucinations
- Sleep problems

Doctors may use:
✔ Antidepressants
✔ Low-dose antipsychotics (very carefully)
✔ Sleep medications
✔ Anti-anxiety drugs

⚠Caution: Some antipsychotics can **worsen confusion**, especially in Lewy body dementia — a reason accurate diagnosis is critical.

✅4. Cognitive and Memory Therapies

Medication is only one part. Therapies help keep the brain active and functional.

Cognitive stimulation therapy (CST):

- Memory games
- Puzzles
- Music therapy
- Reminiscence therapy

- Social engagement

Benefits:
✅Slows decline
✅Improves communication
✅Boosts mood
✅Prevents isolation

✅5. Occupational Therapy

Therapists help patients adapt daily life:

- Dressing
- Bathing
- Eating
- Cooking
- Using memory aids
- Preventing falls
- Making the home safe

Goal: Maintain independence as long as possible.

✅6. Speech Therapy

As language declines, speech therapists help with:

- Word recall
- Communication strategies
- Swallowing issues

✅This reduces frustration and dangerous choking risks.

✅Lifestyle Medicine (Often Ignored but Powerful)

Medical care is not only prescriptions.

Exercise

- Improves blood flow to the brain
- Boosts mood
- Reduces inflammation
- Slows cognitive decline

Even **20–30 minutes daily** makes a difference.

Diet

MIND & Mediterranean diets reduce Alzheimer's risk by **30–53%** in studies.

✔ Leafy greens
✔ Berries
✔ Olive oil
✔ Whole grains
✔ Fish
✔ Nuts
✔ Beans

Heavy sugar and processed food → speeds brain aging

Sleep

Poor sleep increases amyloid buildup.
Good sleep helps the brain clean toxins.

Aim for 7–8 hours nightly.

✅ **Safety and Home Modifications**

Alzheimer's patients are at higher risk of:

- Falls
- Wandering
- Accidents

- Forgetting stoves
- Medication errors

Medical care includes:

✔ Locks on doors
✔ Removing tripping hazards
✔ GPS bracelet for wandering
✔ Medication boxes
✔ Labels on rooms
✔ Night lights

These prevent emergencies and hospitalizations.

✅ **Caregiver Training (Critical but Overlooked)**

Most Alzheimer's care happens **at home**, not in hospitals.

Caregivers need:

- Communication strategies
- Calm de-escalation techniques
- Routines and structure
- Bathing and hygiene skills
- Emergency planning
- Stress management

A trained caregiver reduces:
✅ aggression
✅ anxiety
✅ hospital visits
✅ burnout
✅ patient suffering

✅ **Psychological Care**

Both patient **and family** need emotional support.

- Counseling
- Support groups
- Respite care
- Social activities
- Adult day programs

✅ Loneliness speeds decline
✅ Meaningful activity preserves dignity

✅ Legal & Financial Planning

Alzheimer's eventually affects decision-making.

Planning early protects the family from crisis:

✔ Power of Attorney
✔ Advance medical directives
✔ Will or trust
✔ Financial planning
✔ Long-term care insurance

Families who wait too long often face legal obstacles.

✅ A Chart: Medical Care Checklist

Stage	Main Focus
Early	Diagnosis, medications, lifestyle changes, planning
Middle	Safety, behavior management, caregiver support
Late	Comfort care, infection prevention, hospice support

✅ Common Mistakes Families Make

Mistake	Why It's Dangerous
Waiting too long for	Misses early treatment

Mistake	Why It's Dangerous
diagnosis	window
Skipping medications	Faster decline, more behavior issues
Treating only symptoms, not safety	Risk of injury or wandering
Assuming "nothing can be done"	Leads to rapid deterioration
Ignoring caregiver stress	Leads to abuse, burnout, hospitalization

✅ **Myth-Busting**

❌ **Myth: "Treatment is pointless since there's no cure."**

✅ Treatment can give YEARS of better function.

❌ **Myth: "Medication is enough."**

✅ Without routines, therapy, safety plans, and caregiver support — decline is faster.

❌ **Myth: "Once diagnosed, it's over."**

✅ Many with early Alzheimer's still drive, cook, socialize, travel, and enjoy life.

✅ **Pro Tips for Families**

✔ Start treatment **as early as possible**
✔ Ask about **combination therapy** (meds + lifestyle + therapy)
✔ Build routines — same meals, time, environment
✔ Keep the brain active — music, conversation, activities
✔ Monitor **sleep**, dehydration, depression — they worsen memory
✔ Do not suddenly stop medication without a doctor

✔ Join caregiver support groups
✔ Track behavior changes for doctor visits

✅ The Real Purpose of Alzheimer's Medical Care

Not just to **extend life** —
but to **protect dignity**, reduce suffering, and keep families connected as long as possible.

Medical care helps a person:
✅ recognize loved ones longer
✅ stay safe at home longer
✅ maintain independence longer
✅ reduce emotional distress
✅ enjoy daily life

Even without a cure, **there is hope in good care.**

Table of Contents

www.ingramcontent.com/pod-product-compliance
Lightning Source LLC
LaVergne TN
LVHW011632200926
848484LV00010B/2533